PRAISE FOR

Slow Dancing with a Stranger

"Riveting and necessary."

—*New York Times*

"Comer offers an unflinching and intimate account about what it means to surrender one's career to care for a stricken loved one and conveys a sense of passion and even frustration with a society that she believes has been slow to acknowledge the spread of Alzheimer's disease or make adequate provisions to tend to its caregivers."

—*The Washington Post*

"Poignant, unflinching. . . . [Comer's] memoir is deeply personal and all the more powerful for it."

—*The Miami Herald*

"A cry from the heart of Meryl Comer calls us to confront the scourge of our generation. Alzheimer's disease is laid bare as a slow killer of the health and spirit of the caregiver—the secondary victim, who sacrifices her career and identity to care for a loved one who is lost but still here. Comer's pain is contained in elegant writing and finally channeled into a worthy purpose. But we cannot forget the human cost. Read and recommend this book as a call to action as haunting and urgent as Rachel Carson's *Silent Spring*."

—GAIL SHEEHY,
author of *Passages in Caregiving* and *Daring: My Passages: A Memoir*

"In an unvarnished account of caring for a husband with dementia, Meryl Comer lays out the struggles and gallantry of a devoted and remarkable caregiver."

—PETER RABINS, M.D., MPH,
Professor of Psychiatry and Behavioral Sciences, Johns
Hopkins School of Medicine and author of *The 36-Hour Day*

"No silver linings, no phony homages to 'spiritual growth.' Meryl Comer in *Slow Dancing with a Stranger* writes the unvarnished reality of being exposed as a wife, daughter, caregiver, and potential Alzheimer's victim herself. Admire her bravery and honesty and applaud her for taking away some of the loneliness of the long distance caregiver."

—ELLEN GOODMAN,
Pulitzer Prize–winning, nationally syndicated columnist and
author of *Turning Points*, *Value Judgments*, and *Paper Trail:
Common Sense in Uncommon Times*

"*Slow Dancing with a Stranger* is a remarkable and moving story that will change the way our generation thinks about how we deal with aging and caring for those we love. An amazing journey of caring, love, and resilience."

—TOM RATH,
New York Times bestselling author of *StrengthsFinder 2.0*, *How Full
Is Your Bucket?*, *Strengths Based Leadership*, and *Eat Move Sleep*

"Meryl Comer in *Slow Dancing with a Stranger* unveils Alzheimer's Disease in a remarkable and vulnerable way. Her personal story provides knowledge, inspiration, and hope to us all. Her heroism jumps out from the pages and hopefully will motivate generations to make a difference against this horrible disease."

—DAVID B. AGUS, M.D.,
Professor of Medicine and Engineering, University of
Southern California and author of *The End of Illness* and
A Short Guide to a Long Life

"Meryl Comer was the recipient of the Sargent and Eunice Shriver Profiles in Dignity Award in 2004 for her work as a dedicated advocate and remarkable, decade-long caregiver to her husband with early-onset Alzheimer's. Fast forward a decade later. In *Slow Dancing with a Stranger*, Meryl shows what it truly means to stay the course."

—MARK K. SHRIVER,
Senior Vice President, Save the Children and author of
A Good Man: Rediscovering My Father, Sargent Shriver

"Meryl Comer is a true trailblazer in every aspect of Alzheimer's disease, from nearly twenty years of personal experience in caregiving to leading some of the most exciting and innovative programs for raising public awareness. Her spirit shines through in this exceptional new book chronicling her long and winding journey with this devastating disease."

—DR. RUDY TANZI,
New York Times bestselling author of *Super Brain* and
Joseph P. and Rose F. Kennedy Professor of Neurology,
Massachusetts General Hospital and Harvard Medical School

"*Slow Dancing with a Stranger* is the story of how Meryl Comer became an Alzheimer's caregiver . . . with no warning, no specific training, and no choice. Read this book to understand Alzheimer's but cherish it for the story it is, and you will find that every page breathes with her courage."

—BARRY PETERSEN,
CBS News Correspondent and author of *Jan's Story:
Love Lost to the Long Goodbye of Alzheimer's*

"With her trademark honesty and class, Meryl Comer shares her struggles and triumphs in dealing with Alzheimer's, one of life's most devastating diseases. In *Slow Dancing with a Stranger*, she charts paths that others can follow and recharges the public conversation about a pending global epidemic."

"Meryl Comer's heart-wrenching story will resonate with the millions of families who know the devastation of Alzheimer's disease firsthand. Her journey makes a powerful and compelling case for the urgent need to support Alzheimer's prevention trials."

"This poignant and compelling book is a wake-up call to how Alzheimer's disease can blindside and destroy our efforts to 'age-proof' our lives. Written with great insight and tenderness, *Slow Dancing with a Stranger* is both a cautionary tale and a call to arms as Meryl Comer helps lead the charge to beat this horrific disease before it beats us."

"Meryl Comer is one of my heroes. With unflinching courage, candor, and determination, she eloquently underscores the terrible toll that Alzheimer's takes on patients and families and the urgent need for us to address this unacceptable problem once and for all."

"*Slow Dancing with a Stranger* is a poignant story of Alzheimer's disease robbing memory, personality, life, and dignity. It is an astonishing testimony of a determined woman who decided to fight this disease and to mobilize the world to come up with a cure, a battle to which we all must contribute and win for our parents, ourselves, and future generations.

—PROFESSOR DR. ANDREA PFEIFER,
CEO of AC Immune

"As a physician-scientist who has studied Alzheimer's Disease for more than twenty-five years, and a son with a 99-year-old mom with Alzheimer's dementia, I recommend this book to anyone who is struggling with the tormenting issues of Alzheimer's care."

—MICHAEL E. WIENER, M.D.,
ADNI Principal Investigator and Professor of Medicine,
Radiology, Psychiatry, and Neurology at the University of
California, San Francisco

"Meryl Comer's account of her family's struggle with Alzheimer's is a page-turner; it is wrenching, soul-baring, and beautifully written. It should shock the nation into providing more support—both for Alzheimer's research and treatments and for the legions of family caregivers who will bear ever-growing burdens in the future."

—SUSAN DENTZER,
Senior Policy Adviser to the Robert Wood Johnson Foundation

"Meryl Comer's *Slow Dancing with a Stranger* takes us into the tragedy that is Alzheimer's disease and shows what is ahead for nearly half of us who live to age 85. We must respond to this emergency and Meryl courageously shows us why."

—JEFFREY CUMMINGS, M.D., SCD,
Director of the Cleveland Clinic Lou Ruvo
Center for Brain Health and
KATE ZHONG, M.D.,
Senior Director for Research

"In *Slow Dancing with a Stranger*, Meryl Comer shows us how to acknowledge and endure what on first blush is not endurable, a family afflicted with Alzheimer's. Although she would say she doesn't deserve the recognition, she definitely deserves the 'Rock Star of Humanity' award for her caregiving and her humanitarian work."

—FLORENCE HASELTINE,
Emerita Scientist NIH and Founder of the
Society for Women's Health Research

"Turning tragedy into art and productive work is a hallmark of the great human spirit as it continually turns from the past to give back to the future. Meryl has done this in a very emotional, engaging and thoughtful manner. The book should be read by all, but especially those with Alzheimer's disease in their lives."

—HOWARD FILLIT, M.D.,
Executive Director and Chief Science Officer,
The Alzheimer's Drug Discovery Foundation

"*Slow Dancing with a Stranger* is an unsparing and moving account of the symptoms of early Alzheimer's disease and at the same time a call to arms, a memoir, and an accurate clinical description, deserving a place in the clinical literature on Alzheimer's disease. The author's account will help open readers' minds to the need for early diagnosis of this devastating global illness."

—MARIA ISAAC, M.D., PH.D.,
Psychiatrist, Senior Scientific Officer,
European Medicines Agency

"*Slow Dancing with a Stranger* is a gripping account of the real world issues that the loved ones of Alzheimer's disease families will face and how the community-wide networks of service needed to help any of us cope with this awful disease are woefully inadequate. This a MUST-read for students, service providers, support groups, clergy and policy makers—a primer in why their best intentions too often fail."

—LARRY MINNIX,
President and CEO of LeadingAge

"*Slow Dancing with a Stranger* relates in very human terms the essence of palliative care. Not only did the author care for her husband with unconditional love, but optimized whatever physical and mental capacities were left to preserve his dignity. Readers will be inspired to want to help both victims and caregivers."

—ELIZABETH J. MCCORMACK,
Chairman, Partnership for Palliative Care

"Meryl Comer has courageously penned a heartbreaking open letter from the front lines of caring for a loved one. In a style riveting, candid, powerful, and intimate, Meryl reminds us of the quiet daily heroism of caregivers—and why we must do more to support them."

STACY PAGOS HALLER,
President and Chief Executive Officer,
BrightFocus Foundation

"Meryl Comer has written an amazingly touching, brave, and personal account of her husband's losing battle with Alzheimer's. Her style of advocacy speaks to the power of 'flipping the pain' and deploying the latest digital technologies in fighting an incurable disease."

BARRY LIBERT,
CEO OpenMatters
Strategic Advisor, Angel Investor

"I think there's a mythology that Alzheimer's is a passive fading away of an individual. Nancy Reagan gave us the romantic vision of the long goodbye. Meryl's book highlights the harsh reality. It highlights in a personal way the real story, the impact of the disease not just on the victim but on the entire family. It highlights the need to regard the caregiver as the secondhand victim of the disease."

—GEORGE VRADENBURG,
chairman and founding board member of
UsAgainstAlzheimer's

"This story is real. Meryl and Harvey are real. I don't know what it's going to take to wake the public up to this emerging catastrophe, but I suspect that emotional honesty is a key ingredient. Thank you, Meryl Comer, for telling it exactly like it is."

—DAVID SHENK,
author of *The Forgetting* and creator of the Living with Alzheimer's Film Project

"A poignant love story with a powerful message."

—*Kirkus*

Slow Dancing

WITH A

Stranger

LOST AND FOUND IN THE
AGE OF ALZHEIMER'S

MERYL COMER

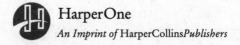

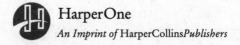
HarperOne
An Imprint of HarperCollinsPublishers

HarperOne

HarperCollins books may be purchased for educational, business, or sales promotional use. For information please e-mail the Special Markets Department at SPsales@harpercollins.com.

HarperCollins website: http://www.harpercollins.com

HarperCollins®, 🏭®, and HarperOne™ are trademarks of HarperCollins Publishers.

FIRST HARPERCOLLINS PAPERBACK EDITION PUBLISHED IN 2015

Designed by Janet M. Evans

Library of Congress Cataloging-in-Publication Data

Comer, Meryl.
      Slow dancing with a stranger : lost and found in the age of
   Alzheimer's / Meryl Comer. — First edition.
         pages cm
      ISBN 978–0–06–213085–3
      1. Alzheimer's disease—Patients—Biography. 2. Alzheimer's
   disease—Patients—Family relationships—Biography. 3. Caregivers—
   Biography. 4. Physicians—Diseases—Biography. I. Title.
   RC523.C656   2014
   362.1968'31—dc23   2014001630

15 16 17 18 19   RRD(H)   10 9 8 7 6 5 4 3 2 1

To Hope, Eli, and Benjamin:

May your memories last a lifetime.

Contents

EVERY 68 SECONDS

The man I live with is not the man I fell in love with and married.

He has slowly been robbed of something we all take for granted: the ability to navigate the mundane activities of daily living—bathing, shaving, dressing, feeding, and using the bathroom. His inner clock is confused and can't be reset. His eyes are vacant and unaware—as if an internal window shade veils our access.

Before I grasped what was happening, I was hurt and annoyed by my husband's behavior. Those feelings dissolved into unconditional empathy once I understood the cruelty of his diagnosis: early-onset Alzheimer's disease. He was fifty-eight.

At first, I ran interference and fought for him because it was the right thing to do. He was slipping out of control—confused, childlike and helpless, his social filters stripped away. He shadowed me because I was familiar and safe, even when he could no longer remember my name.

I always loved him, but during our marriage, he was often aloof and unreachable. In illness, unlike in health, he made me feel needed and important to him.

Neither a scientist nor a neurologist, I have spent close to two decades trying to decipher what's going on in my husband's head. How hard and unfair it is for such a smart man to lose pieces of his intellect and independence as the circuitry of his brain misfires and corrodes. No new short-term memories stick: his internal navigational compass has shut down. His disease is my crossword puzzle.

Harvey has long forgotten me, but I am constant as his copilot and guardian. Every conversation is inclusive and respectful even though he is often unintelligible or mute. It is a charade that never ends. I bear the burden of all decisions for us both. The demons and terror of his world define mine. Any challenge is self-defeating. I play into his reality and pretend that his fate and our life together are not doomed. Unfortunately, I know better.

Alzheimer's distorts and destroys shared memories that bind family ties. Caregivers are not unlike victims who survive a hurricane and find ourselves sifting through the rubble to rescue faded, storm-drenched photos or sentimental objects. We piece together what's left of our past and struggle to put down building blocks for the future. I need to make some sense of my journey through this storm.

My bookshelf is lined with tomes on dementia care, yet the page I need always seems to be missing. Each brain unravels in its own quirky and idiosyncratic way. I have learned first-hand that there is no single solution to taking care of someone with dementia.

Many times, personal stories involving Alzheimer's gloss over the unseemly details of care. They are written as love stories of unquestioned devotion or living memorials to honor someone during better times. Why not? As spouses and caregivers, we deserve to do whatever works for us. It is our version of pain management. But I never wanted to embellish or soften the edges around the truth. It does not do justice to the cruelty of the disease. I offer you my own experiences from a position of hard-won humility. I hope you will thread them with your own.

When I say I have cared full-time for Harvey in our home all these years, many ask me why. Even now, there is always an initial reflex that makes me want to say, "Do I really need to explain myself after all I've been through?"

I realize that the question is a natural one, a human one, a social one. The interlocutors are not judging me, but rather vicariously checking themselves. In questioning me, they are testing their own capacity to deal with a diagnosis of Alzheimer's disease and the potential impact it might have on their relationship with a partner or parent.

When people hear my story, they sometimes tell me they wouldn't make the same choices. I do not hold myself up as an example to follow. No one who has been on the frontlines of care ever questions when someone says "I can't do this anymore." But I do want to be part of the last generation of caregivers trapped by a loved one's diagnosis, an absence of disease-modifying therapies, and a troublesome lack of quality care options.

When it comes to Alzheimer's, caregivers are frequently too worn out or isolated to protest. Perhaps this is why advocacy around the disease has often lacked the passion and energy that characterize the cancer and HIV communities. But how will people understand if we do not tell our stories without apology?

Alzheimer's disease today affects a reported 5.4 million people in the United States and 44 million worldwide. Like a stealth invader, it is quietly dementing aging populations globally while quickly pushing past cancer and HIV/AIDS as the most critical public health problem of our time. Every 68 seconds, another of us falls victim. Yet, fifty percent of those with dementia never get diagnosed.

My greatest fear is that mine will be the family next door by mid-century.

There is not a single FDA-approved drug that actually slows the progression of Alzheimer's disease. There have been too many failed late-stage clinical trials with promising drugs that seemed to work—until it became clear they did not.

Sometimes I think we would be better off if Alzheimer's disease was a brand-new emergency instead of a century-old threat to which we somehow have become inured. Perhaps people would understand that when it comes to this disease, everyone is a stakeholder, because everyone is at risk.

There are also 15 million caregivers just like me; unintended victims and not among the official count. Add to our legions those caring for loved ones—young and old—with diseases of the brain, traumatic brain injuries, and other chronic diseases complicated by a memory disorder. We speak the same language. Our numbers amplify the collective pain that makes it impossible for me to rest.

The only way to minimize the effects of Alzheimer's disease is to get out in front of it; delay its onset or even reverse its devastation of the mind. We need to move toward early diagnosis and study adults who do not yet show symptoms. People like you and me.

Such a decision entails hard personal choices, risks, and emotional discomfort. It means demanding safe and clinically valid genetic tests that let us learn if we are at higher risk for getting Alzheimer's disease. It requires managing our lives and choices under the shadow of the possibility of disease.

Those of us who are fifty years and older must stop viewing ourselves as ageless. All of us should track our cognitive health, just as we do cholesterol levels or blood pressure. We need to overcome fear and stop cowering in the shadows of stigma.

I write for all of us who are still well, but have seen the devastation of Alzheimer's disease firsthand. The emergency is with us and in us.

I write to clinicians, reluctant to diagnose because they can't effectively treat. Please know the inadvertent trauma you inflict on families left confused, hurt, and helpless. Then time runs out on the ultimate conversation with our loved ones about end-of-life wishes. Their minds are erased. It is simply too late.

I write to reach the generation of our adult sons and daughters, who struggle to understand our lives as we care for a loved one with Alzheimer's. They stand on the precipice and wrestle with issues and decisions similar to the ones we have faced. They deserve better options and not the bankrupting burden of our care. This is not the legacy we want for our children or the way anyone wishes to be remembered.

I write for my grandchildren because, no matter how hard I tried, Alzheimer's blanketed my home with sadness. I know that loving each of them unconditionally has been my salvation. One day, I hope they read these words and appreciate my choices.

As I write these words, a faint glow fills the room I share with Harvey. He is always present, even though he is absent. There is an intimacy in our isolation. Nonetheless, I am willing to open the door to our room in the hope that you will find a way inside. Only then will my story be worth the pain of its telling.

ONE

EARLY SIGNS

This is not the first time I have sat staring at the computer screen wondering how to begin or what to say. As a former TV news reporter, I know how to write succinctly about complex issues. I spent most of my career finding ways to allow people to quickly grasp whatever was happening that day.

Perhaps what stops me is a feeling I cannot shake—that it is premature, even emotionally offensive, to write an obituary while he is still alive. We do it all the time in network news, whenever a notable is seriously ill. That way, we are ready when the time comes to break the sad headlines with a touching tribute that invites us all to share vicarious memories. But in this case, who really cares?—except our immediate family, who also lives in limbo. The man I knew, loved, and married has been absent and anonymous for years, even though he lives at home and is cared for by me. Close friends and coworkers abandoned us long ago. It was too disconcerting to walk through our door and see someone who was once just like them being destroyed in slow motion by an insidious disease for which there is no cure. I understand how they feel, even though I was left behind too and I'm not sick. How do I write about a twenty-year gaping hole in our lives—an intimate part of our history—when it's still not over?

I am not sure when people at work realized that something was wrong with Harvey. But I remember vividly how his behavior at home changed.

This commanding, strong-willed, yet considerate man became upset when things didn't go his way. The slightest thing set him off. If he couldn't find his wallet, keys, or papers, accusations flew that someone, anyone at home but Harvey, had taken them. When I mentioned the change in his behavior, he erupted in anger. In the face of his wrath, I went silent, infuriating him even more. These episodes usually ended with Harvey storming out, slamming the front door and driving off. It was painful, and I wondered if our marriage was in trouble.

Now I know that this behavior is common in the early stages of the disease, when symptoms are emerging but not yet full blown. The Academy of Neurology reports that the pressures on family life due to Alzheimer's begin long before active dementia is apparent, and this was my experience too. Individuals start to privately fight the earliest stages of dementia but are unable to articulate what is wrong. The stress on them and their loved ones is overwhelming.

It is impossible to detect exactly when this process starts, and it was especially difficult in the case of someone like Harvey. He was the type of person who always got noticed. When he walked in the room, you knew he was there.

At the National Institutes of Health, where he had worked since the 1960s, most of the male scientists wore khakis, a wrinkled non-iron shirt, and a blue blazer to work every day. Harvey was always impeccably dressed in the latest styles. As a high school student, he had worked in a men's clothing shop to earn extra money, and his father never let him spend the cash on clothes. Harvey made up for lost time as an adult. Most days, he had to wear a white lab coat but still managed to assert his sartorial taste with English cuffed shirts, French silk ties, and the most flamboyant socks peeking above his soft Italian suede or leather loafers.

Harvey was on the international scientific circuit and traveled frequently to Europe to attend conferences and present papers. He always returned home with a refrigerated box containing medical samples and, tucked amid the dry ice, tins of foie gras, Petrossian caviar, and smoked salmon from Fauchon, a gourmet food shop on the right bank of the Seine. His suitcase was a gourmand's treasure trove: boxes of Richart handmade chocolate, macarons from Ladurée on the Champs-Élysées, and at least two or three bottles of wine wrapped in his clothes. There were new ties, the old ones stained purple from a tasting tour in Burgundy or Bordeaux—his rationale for indulging himself with even more ties. He drove a canary yellow 911 Porsche to work every day, which he enjoyed so much that I not so jokingly referred to it as his mistress. It glimmered in the parking lot at the NIH, a foreign traveler in a land where most of the other cars were sensible four-door sedans. In the evenings, after a long day caring for patients or working in the lab, he liked to hit the gas pedal. I could hear the distinctive engine roar a block away as he entered our street—a ten-minute route he drove for thirty-one years, until the disease impaired his ability to find his way home.

From the beginning, Harvey and I used to joke that it was amazing we found each other. He had a son, Mark, from a first marriage that ended in divorce. His second wife left unannounced one day, taking everything with her. It left him bitter and untrusting. I was a single mother with a five-year-old son. I rarely had time or inclination to socialize, but one day a neighbor asked me to drop by her house on a Sunday afternoon to meet an eligible doctor friend who was there to watch a football game. At first I demurred, but she persisted. I gave in but told her I was coming with my son and wasn't going to put on makeup.

It has been almost forty years since the day we met, and even now I remember every detail. Harvey, long and lean, was dressed in a forest green wool turtleneck, corduroy slacks, and well-worn hiking boots. He was more distinguished looking than handsome, but it was hard to ignore his steely blue eyes. He was smoking a hand-carved Algerian briar pipe that wafted a woodsy aroma of Dunhill #6. Jason and I arrived at the house during a dramatic fourth-quarter play between the New York Giants and the Green Bay Packers, and Harvey, a Giants fan, was distracted. He invited Jason to sit next to him on the couch. The image of the two of them sitting companionably together gave me a sharp pang of longing. This was what I wanted: a father for my son and a family life. Confused by my feelings, I retreated to the kitchen. My five-year-old was the one who invited Harvey to come over to our house.

For our first date a week later, we agreed that Harvey would stop by after I returned home from anchoring the ten o'clock news. He arrived shortly after the sitter left, and Jason was already sound asleep. I headed for the kitchen to get him a drink while he settled onto my couch. When I returned less than five minutes later, he was sound asleep, having started his day at the hospital around six in the morning. I tried to wake him, but he didn't budge. So I grabbed a throw blanket, draped it over him, turned off the lights, and went up to bed. When I came down in the morning, he was gone. No note—just gone.

Later, we joked that a relationship would never work. We had very different lives. Despite the uncertainty, neither of us wanted to end things. Then something happened that crystallized for me why. Four months into our relationship, I got a call late one afternoon, just two weeks before Jason and I were to join my mother for my brother Steve's graduation from Antioch College. It was the local police saying that my brother had been reported missing and later found in a wooded area near campus, dead of a self-inflicted gunshot wound to the head. The police needed me to identify the body. I didn't want to disturb Harvey at work for fear of asking too much from a new relationship. I left a brief voice message saying that I had to go out of town unexpectedly. I was packing to leave when Harvey showed up at the front door. He offered to stay with Jason or come with me to help. Three days later, my brother was buried under a tree, next to the red stable where he used to teach children with physical disabilities to ride. I emptied out his apartment, packed a truck with his things, and adopted his mongrel dog, Sash, whom he had left behind with extra food, water, and a note. "I can't lock my heart away in a box for safekeeping," he wrote, referring to a love affair gone sour, as we mourned our loss. My mother flew back to Washington alone. Harvey showed up with a cooler under his arm, and we drove back in the truck. He said he didn't want me to go it alone. Six months later, he moved in with us.

Four years later, we were married in the empty living room of an old Spanish-style home we bought together and planned to renovate. We invited thirty guests, including the neighbor who had introduced us. Harvey showed up late to his own wedding; he was tending to a very sick patient at the NIH.

The truth is that Harvey's research and his patients took precedence throughout our marriage. I grew used to him missing holidays, canceling vacations, and rescheduling dinner with friends. He was not generous with expressions of love, which is one reason I treasured a letter he wrote to me aboard a night flight to Paris shortly after we met. Tucked behind a fading, yet favorite photo and the last one of Harvey well, it read: "Dearest M,"—M was his nickname for me—"I miss you terribly and I am only 2½ hours away from you. I am not sure that I express my true feelings to you, but the inner euphoria and excitement is something I have never experienced before. The seat next to me is empty, and I have turned to it hoping that somehow you will be there."

Given our work and travel schedules, our favorite times were the weekends, when we stayed home and read the Sunday *New York Times* together. When we did go out in the evening, Harvey always took charge of ordering the wine. In a French restaurant, he spoke to the waiters in excellent French, which he taught himself by listening to Foreign Service language tapes while out for his daily long-distance run. It was one thing we did together with our dog, Sash, whom Harvey spoiled and from whom he got unconditional love in return. Our six-mile runs didn't exactly promote togetherness, though. Harvey was always two hundred yards ahead of me, mesmerized in his next language lesson or deep in thought about an experiment that hadn't lived up to his expectations.

Many of his personal interests and passions grew out of a two-year medical sabbatical that he spent in Paris in the early 1980s, just one year after we married. Jason and I were invited to go along, but at the time I had just worked my way back on TV with a business show and Jason was busy with school. I never wanted to rely on Harvey financially and needed to work. We split expenses right down the middle on everything, including vacations. I worried that when his sabbatical was over, I would be unable to find another job.

Our friends were shocked that we would even consider living apart so soon after marrying. To Harvey, they said, "How can you leave your new wife? Didn't you learn anything from the demise of your second marriage?" To me, they demanded, "How can you let your husband go off to Paris alone when he won't even wear a wedding ring?" We plunged ahead, agreeing to be a commuting couple.

Solo in Paris, Harvey learned to love wine and began buying futures in 1982 Bordeaux, Burgundy, and Champagne. This indulgence on a researcher's salary was made possible by a strong international currency market and a dollar at its highest in decades against the franc. It also helped that I was his silent partner and gave him carte blanche. He also bought himself a raven-blue BMW, which he kept in a garage in a small residential neighborhood alongside the Seine in the 16th arrondissement.

During the day, he walked for miles, exploring the alleyways and side streets, stopping for a cup of coffee or a glass of wine. He was always looking to duck into an interesting store and chat with the owner or strike up a conversation with someone walking down the street. He usually ended with dinner at a family-run restaurant where the owner cooked him her specialties. On weekends, he got the car out, took to the autoroute, and detoured off through the countryside to visit the vineyards. He eagerly tasted the wine, asked questions, and learned to distinguish the subtle differences that made one vintage more valuable than another.

A shrewd man, he built our wine collection the way he played the stock market, looking for a promising but overlooked wine whose value might grow in time. He bought first growths relatively cheap, shipped the crates to a U.S. distributor, and then stored the bottles in a specially built cellar with its own cooling system.

Two years went by relatively quickly, and when Harvey returned back to the United States, it was his wine obsession and not a desire to improve my closet space that prompted our home renovation. I purposely turned a blind eye to our growing liquid investment. Such a perishable asset made me nervous, but it gave him great pleasure and a diversion from work. The wine cellar was the place Harvey retreated to decompress after a long day at work. He liked to spend an uninterrupted hour there turning the bottles and checking the air temperature and humidity. With such precise attention to detail, one would think that there would be wine journals with meticulous records, but Harvey wrote little down and kept the base prices in his head. Was it the arrogance we all share that our minds won't fail us? If he found one bottle with a bad cork, it became an excuse to throw an impromptu dinner party with wine tasting as the centerpiece of conversation.

At heart, we were homebodies comfortable with each other and a few close friends who tolerated that we both worked ungodly hours—I was out the door at 3:00 A.M. to prepare for a morning newscast and he was in the hospital by six. We dressed and partied only when professionally obligated to make an appearance, and usually attended separate events, he going to gatherings with scientists and his NIH colleagues and I with my friends and colleagues in the media and business world.

In this way, we were not unlike many working couples who have separate professional acquaintances and a small cadre of friends shared in common. And yet, this very dynamic kept me from realizing that the issues I started noticing at home were being mirrored on the job.

At work, his colleagues assumed his behavior might be related to personal problems at home, while I wondered if the changes in mood were due to pressures at work. This situation is not uncommon in early-onset cases. These cases don't fit the face of Alzheimer's: too young, too physically fit, and too self-aware for anyone to realize that something is not quite right. Work that was routine becomes exhausting because the disease infiltrates and destroys the neural connections responsible for executive function in the brain. The hippocampus goes into overdrive, and the process of hiding out begins.

Where Harvey most closely fit the stereotype of the brilliant but eccentric scientist was the way he maintained his office. Sometimes people walked by just to take a look. Most days, it was impossible to enter. People poked their heads in, stunned to see the floor completely covered with papers and documents. Books, charts for his latest paper, the most recent journals opened haphazardly to a piece he was reading, all of it piled in towers that teetered, threatening to crash at any moment if someone got too close. Amid this chaos, Harvey ruled, propelled by a remarkable ability to remember exactly where everything was located. Despite the apparent lack of order, until he got sick, he was always able to retrieve from the pile the single article he needed to make a point.

I rarely visited his office—he had patients and his research to tend to—but when I did, I was absolutely mortified by what I saw. Harvey was a man so exacting about his research that he used himself as a control in experiments. Yet he worked in an office that looked like robbers had ransacked it. I could never tell Harvey what to do, so I just suggested he keep his office door shut when he wasn't there.

An early sign that something was amiss came during one of my infrequent visits to his office, as I watched him struggle unsuccessfully to find something in the piles of documents.

Unread periodicals and untouched newspapers that he had once devoured started stacking up at home, as his ability to concentrate for extended periods waned. Struggling to maintain control, Harvey made such a financial mess that it took me four years to clean up our accounts. Second marriages typically mean separate bank accounts, which mitigated some of the damage. But even now, I still find outdated checks that were never cashed and documents squirreled away in the strangest places from his paranoid days.

The latest research supports the idea that one of the first signs of dementia is a change in behavior. If someone has always forgotten names, then forgetting names is not necessarily a sign of dementia. Rather, it is a decline in one's typical abilities, a change from the usual behavior. It was not the lack of order in Harvey's office that signaled problems. Rather, it was Harvey looking around his office in confusion, overwhelmed by the chaos that had never fazed him before, which signaled that something was going terribly wrong.

He had a reputation at work of being brilliant but sometimes prickly, and later many of his colleagues cited his personality quirks as one reason it took so long to notice his decline. At the beginning of his illness, his moodiness just seemed like a more intense version of the way he sometimes was, moving quickly between charm and impatience. When he wanted to persuade someone, he could be the most engaging man in the room, animated and charismatic. He smiled often, telling jokes or making clever remarks. There was an art to the way he moved, filling the room with his intellect and personality, putting his hand on someone's shoulder to suggest complicity in whatever he was saying. He had a way of making people feel that they were part of his team; that they were all in the fight together. But when someone disagreed with him and he didn't think they had made a good case, he could make a cutting remark that stung. Not everyone could keep up with his rapid train of thought, his depth of knowledge—which came from years of studying the smallest details of what made one leukemia different from another—or his fiercely worded arguments.

In a debate over patient care, Harvey was formidable and rarely gave in once he had made up his mind about what to do. A colleague once remarked that if you wanted to change an order that Harvey had given, you had to go into the meeting prepared for a fight. Harvey rarely gave in.

As time went on and the disease slowly progressed, changes in Harvey's behavior became noticeable. When they pressed him to give his opinion, he faltered. He had trouble remembering clinical details they had just told him a few minutes before or he gave answers that were irrelevant to the discussion. One time when someone asked him about the level of potassium in a patient, Harvey started talking instead about vitamin K—*K* is the chemical symbol for potassium, which is totally different from the vitamin. The fellows started to suspect that something was wrong.

Word that something was amiss with Harvey eventually reached the more senior doctors. One doctor said he dismissed the reports at first, saying he hadn't noticed any changes and that the novice doctor must have caught the department chief on a bad day. But as more reports of Harvey losing his train of thought started to circulate, his colleagues started paying closer attention. At the beginning, most of them assumed stress at home or some professional frustration. They also considered depression or an adverse reaction to a medication.

One day, I got a call from Henry Masur, NIH chief of critical care, who worked with Harvey. People were starting to talk, he told me. Harvey seemed distracted at work. He couldn't concentrate. He started sentences but then trailed off, as if he had lost his train of thought. Masur told me that he had confronted Harvey about it earlier in the week and asked him what was going on, if he was taking any medications that might be affecting his cognitive abilities, if something was happening in his personal life that might be making it harder to concentrate at work.

I was both distraught and relieved by the call. I had watched Harvey's personality shift in small, incremental ways. At first, I assumed that he was able to pull himself together at work. After all, being with patients was Harvey's lifeblood. He was the type of doctor who was called by pediatrics to give painful spinal taps to children because of his expertise and caring bedside manner. He took the time to explain to patients the goals of his research, and they offered to enroll in trials testing his ideas. When the cutting-edge therapies stopped working, Harvey was the one who went back to the hospital at night with wine and meals I had cooked, to spend time talking with his dying patients.

I always attributed his tenacity and desire to become a doctor to his overwhelming feelings of hopelessness as an only child of two parents who were chronically and seriously ill throughout his youth—a child who walked the mile from school to the hospital to visit them, doing his homework by their bedside, and then when visiting hours were over, making his way back home to let himself into a dark and lonely apartment. By age fourteen, when he broke his arm playing baseball and a doctor fixed it, he had become determined to be a doctor and save lives.

Now I was learning that the scaffolding of Harvey's identity—his work as a doctor—was falling apart. Masur reported to me that when confronted, Harvey responded that lately he was not feeling well and he had already been to the doctor. This wasn't true. Harvey continued to refuse my entreaties that he see a doctor. His personality was also shifting from type A in overdrive to something more aggressive, egocentric, and emotionally abusive. It took all Harvey's mental capacity to hold himself together at work, so he exploded at home.

A confrontation at Thanksgiving, pardonable only in hindsight, left a bitter aftertaste in our memories as a family. My son, Jason, brought his fiancée, Dana, to join in an intimate family celebration. The china, silver, and crystal gleamed atop linens specially chosen to match the flower arrangement of giant chrysanthemums. Everything seemed fine, with the conversation polite and low-key. Then we sat down to dinner. Jason offered to assist by carving the turkey, and without warning, Harvey started to yell. Brandishing the carving knife in his hand, Harvey warned Jason not to try to usurp his role as head of the family. Shocked, we sat in stunned silence, unable to move. Then just as suddenly, Harvey dropped the knife on the table and stormed out of the dining room, grabbing the car keys hanging near the door and heading out into the chilly night without a jacket. I let him go. Long after midnight, after everyone else had left, Harvey came home. He never explained what had triggered his extreme behavior, and he offered no apology.

This was the pendulum along which our lives now swung: months of lucidity punctured by sudden, inexplicable rages. I didn't know what to do.

Was my mind playing tricks? Was whatever haunted Harvey also taunting me?

I clung to the notion that things might somehow get better. Instead, they got worse. Six months after the incident at Thanksgiving, the family gathered again, this time for Jason and Dana's rehearsal dinner and wedding. The dinner was held at a popular restaurant selected by my ex-husband. Family and friends had gathered from all over the country to celebrate, and I did not want a repeat of the Thanksgiving fiasco. We all agreed that only Dana's parents, Jason's biological father, and I would offer toasts. Harvey arrived late with Mark, who didn't seem to tune into his dad's subtle, yet erratic behavior. Even though it was mid-March and the room cold, Harvey sweated profusely and refused to make eye contact.

The evening started out smoothly, but no sooner did Dana's father sit down after toasting the bride and groom than Harvey abruptly stood up and started speaking. He spoke forcefully, as he always did when addressing a crowd, but his facial expression was wooden. He stared straight ahead and kept wiping his forehead. Every so often, he suddenly stopped speaking, giving the impression that he was about to sit down. Invariably, he just started talking again.

Not once did Harvey mention the joy of the occasion. Instead, he talked on and on about a distant cousin that he hadn't seen in years and who he learned had just died. The guests listened in stunned silence, unsure of what to make of the strange speech and Harvey's odd behavior.

I finally took action. During one of his short pauses, I stood up and started to applaud, hoping to stop Harvey from continuing to talk. Then I asked everyone to join me in a toast to the new couple. Everyone raised their glass. Harvey sat down stiffly, staring straight ahead. As soon as I could, I went to Jason and Dana to apologize, but it is hard to undo a moment like that.

I stayed behind at the hotel that night to take care of my elderly mother while Harvey and Mark went home. I tried to anticipate how I could intervene if Harvey didn't know where to go after he escorted my mother down the aisle to her seat. Would he remember he had to continue to the front to join the best man? Or would he turn around and walk or do something embarrassing, like address the audience? I barely slept, thinking about how many things might go wrong.

I had brought a backup tux with me in case Harvey did not dress appropriately, and the next morning it came in handy. Harvey arrived at the hotel wearing a regular shirt and tie under the tux jacket, no bow tie, and sporty shoes—another giveaway that the sharp dresser I knew was no more. I helped him dress for the occasion, hoping when he saw himself in the formal clothes, it might remind him of how to act.

At the wedding, Harvey made it down the aisle and through the ceremony. During dinner, I sat next to him, sipping from his wine glass so he would not drink too much and deflecting questions when he seemed confused or unable to answer. Toward the end of the evening, he announced that he was driving Mark to a cousin's home in New Jersey and returning the same night. I begged him not to go, fearing that after he dropped off his son, he might become disoriented and get lost. At 3:00 A.M. frantic that he had not returned, I filed a missing persons report to the New Jersey state police. A few hours later, Harvey walked in the door, disheveled, sweaty, and confused. He said the police caught him speeding on the highway. Then without further discussion, he got into bed with the tux still on and fell asleep.

I didn't want to admit to Masur—or to myself— that these kinds of events were increasingly common. Rightly, he would feel professionally obligated to report everything I said to Harvey's superiors. Harvey's entire life had been spent taking care of others. His research efforts were devoted to offering dying cancer patients more quality of life and more time. Now that he was struggling, didn't he deserve the same consideration? I needed to find out what was wrong and still protect Harvey. When Masur proposed more precise neurological workups and outside experts rather than colleagues running tests, I was on board.

Over the next few weeks, Masur shared a list of possible diagnoses. Harvey was prematurely gray, so some of his colleagues speculated that he might have pernicious anemia. Based on his symptoms, other conditions that came to mind were a brain tumor, Lyme disease, and even mad cow disease from one of his trips to London.

But in all those conversations, one thing we never discussed was Alzheimer's disease. Early-onset cases were not immediately considered in someone only fifty-six years old. I had to learn firsthand that doctors avoid giving an Alzheimer's diagnosis, preferring to first rule out other conditions. Moreover, twenty years ago when Harvey first began showing symptoms,

Alzheimer's was steeped in stigma. People did not like to discuss it. Even for Harvey's colleagues, what was happening didn't make sense. None of it did.

Despite my growing concern and that of his colleagues, it wasn't easy to get Harvey to see a specialist. It is hard enough to get any loved one in the early stages of a disease to see a doctor, especially when the symptoms don't have a specific name or apparent cause. My efforts were hampered by the fact that Harvey had been making clinical decisions for other people all his life and was certain that he could make one for himself. I asked our attorney and close personal friend to persuade Harvey that only a clean bill of health from a neurologist could get them off his back.

I had to talk our way to the front of the line for an appointment with a top neurologist in Washington, D.C., who was about to retire. As a professional courtesy, he agreed to see him. I will never forget that appointment. A doctor's visit that took less than forty-five minutes kept us from being able to get my husband's condition accurately diagnosed for more than two years. The two of them interacted as fellow medical professionals, leaving me as the interloper, a concerned wife who was overreacting. When we arrived at the doctor's office, his citations and awards were packed. What happened next complicated everything. Harvey told him one account of what was going on, and I set out to tell another.

Knowing what I was up against I came prepared, handing them both a typed list of symptoms that I and his colleagues at work had independently observed: high levels of irritability, attention distracted instead of focused, difficulty processing new information, frequent loss of train of thought, tendency to stop midsentence, and inability to recover. Then there were the erratic and unexplained behaviors like getting lost on the short drive to work—a route he had driven for more than twenty-five years—leaving the car running in front of the house to find it stolen when he came out an hour later, having to ask me where to sign a check, imagining that someone was stealing money from his account even when the bank statement matched, and losing endless time shuffling through his research papers. He complained of exhaustion but could not sleep, broke into cold sweats, said he was hungry but forgot to eat, was losing eye-hand coordination when we played tennis, repeatedly asked me the same question (requiring me to pretend it was the first time just to keep the peace).

What I did not write down and would only say when directly questioned by the neurologist was how much these behaviors were taking a toll on our marriage. They were, but Harvey was already agitated by the list of observations, and his cold stare prompted me to say only that the situation was tense. I had already offered numerous examples. Other problems—that he was no longer interested in sex, seemed lost at home, locked himself in the bathroom and couldn't figure his way out—went unmentioned.

The only way to keep Harvey from jumping out of his chair and bolting for the door was to relate everything back to a shared concern that "whatever" was going on with him threatened to dismantle his career. Then the doctor and Harvey disappeared into the examining room for no more than twenty minutes. When they returned, the doctor looked at me, while winking at Harvey, and said, "No need to worry. The examination shows no gross abnormalities. You've upset yourself unnecessarily. Your husband may be suffering from stress and a bit of depression. I have a prescription for the stress, and for the other, I recommend the two of you take a long-overdue vacation." I panicked, knowing that Harvey was scheduled to give an important speech and had a trip to London planned to attend a medical meeting the following week. I desperately needed the doctor to intervene, but he was dismissive. On the way out he said to Harvey, "You're fine. You can do anything you want to do, but lighten up your caseload and have this prescription filled. And little lady, your husband is in great physical shape and knows exactly what he is doing. Get off his back. Time to relax."

I was shocked by the doctor's refusal to respect what I had to say. In presenting the information, I had forced myself to speak in an analytic, almost detached manner, despite my rising panic at what was happening in my own home. Yet I was still being dismissed as some kind of overwrought, anxious spouse. Trying to keep my annoyance in check, I asked for a copy of the examination report before we left. I knew it was just a matter of time before NIH would require documentation that Harvey was still fit to work, and our lawyer would need to officially offer it for Harvey's record. A glance at Harvey's chart showed that my detailed notes plotting the dates of specific changes in behavior were missing. The neurologist had let professional courtesy extend too far. Noted and underlined in the report was the doctor's much more benign conclusion: "No gross abnormalities," along with a prescription for an antipsychotic to treat depression.

As soon as we left the doctor's office with report in hand, Harvey attacked. He warned me not to insult him again. His basic message was that what went on at work was his business and not mine. That fateful encounter left me tiptoeing carefully around Harvey, who grew even more headstrong and obstinate after his escape with a clean bill of health. I knew that Harvey had been on his best behavior with the neurologist and managed to pull it together enough to make it through the examination, but I was certain that eventually the charade would catch up with him.

Unfortunately, it was not a conscious game for Harvey. He was in denial about any deficit, his skill as a diagnostician undermined by the unperceived creep of mild cognitive impairment. Yet he volunteered that he had temporarily taken himself off patient care as a precaution until he felt better. My son's wife, Dana, was working on her master's thesis in social work and interning at NIH. She observed Harvey in the NIH library, staring at his research and then disappearing into the stacks. Dana reported to me that she often walked back with him to his office under the pretense she was headed to the same floor in the Clinical Center.

My work suffered as I tried to keep up with my demanding job while running interference for Harvey. I lived every day anticipating a crisis, running through what-if scenarios before I left in the morning and before I went to sleep at night. It was hard to concentrate on what was happening at work or get excited about new assignments. I jumped each time the phone rang, assuming the worst. There was no time for living in denial with him. I was now the point person for two, with one of the two resisting my efforts every step of the way.

TWO

A DIFFERENT REALITY

A few weeks after the doctor's appointment, my fears were realized. Harvey had been asked to give a major talk on leukemia months earlier. Now that date was suddenly upon us. I begged Harvey not to give the speech. At home, the signs were even more pronounced than they were at work. Buttressed by the identity that had been the framework of his entire life, Harvey still was reasonably cogent when he was with his peers. Even when he could not retain details about a patient's case that someone had told him ten minutes earlier, he was able to look at a slide and talk about the disease. This is how smart people hide out in the early stages of dementia.

But at home he seemed lost. He sat in the chair in our kitchen nook after dinner, frantically sorting through documents related to his research or dumping out his slide deck and starting over. Now he faced the prospect of standing up in front of a room filled with professionals. Speeches given at conferences are an important part of the scientific process. They are meant to be challenged, giving scientists a chance to probe the data and push one another about their theories. I knew Harvey would be fortunate if he made it through the entire speech, let alone handled questions from the audience. Yet the doctor's report from a few weeks earlier silenced me when I should have spoken up. I felt crushed that the doctor had dismissed my concerns but fearful that if I went public, my actions might ruin Harvey's reputation. So I took the middle path. I did not share my concerns, but decided to go with him that day in case something went wrong.

The lecture before four hundred doctors was held in a big ballroom at a hotel in downtown Bethesda, Maryland, not far from where we lived. In the good old days, Harvey typically would run late for such a conference, arriving five minutes before he was going to go on stage but still able to present his slides, data, and conclusions as if he had been preparing for hours. Those days were behind us. I told Harvey that I would drive him. In a sign that should have tipped me off that we should cancel the appearance, Harvey agreed.

The issue of Harvey continuing to drive was an ongoing area of contention between us. Imagine what it was like trying to take a sports car away from a fifty-six-year-old man. The Porsche represented not only a beautiful piece of engineering that gave Harvey pleasure to drive but a symbol of his personal freedom and independence. But as Harvey's symptoms worsened, my worries about him driving grew. In addition to the car being stolen and then recovered, there had already been a number of episodes of lost keys found in the ignition. A few months earlier, an unexplained accident had ended with his Porsche straddling the median strip on the highway. I didn't even learn about it until two days later, when I got a call from a towing company about the charge for extracting the car and taking it to the dealership. Fortunately, no one was hurt, but what shocked me more was that Harvey didn't remember what had happened.

Another time, with my son and his wife watching from the front steps of our house, Harvey got in the car and shifted into gear but forgot what to do next. Instead of backing down the driveway, the car lurched forward in jerking motions. Jason yelled frantically, trying to tell Harvey how to stop. Luckily, the car smashed into a line of tall spruce trees that bordered a high embankment down to the main street. It was the only thing that kept the car from flipping over.

Despite the evidence of the damaged car, Harvey still refused to admit he was having trouble. Many evenings, the short drive from the NIH to our home, a route that Harvey had driven on autopilot for decades, took much longer. When I confronted Harvey, he angrily refused to discuss the matter further.

When I suggested he stop driving, Harvey shut down emotionally. He ignored me or left the room in anger. I started to think that I should get the keys away from him before he seriously hurt himself or someone else, but I was foiled at every turn.

Two weeks earlier, Harvey had gone to the Department of Motor Vehicles to get his license renewed. I was sure he would never pass and the problem would be resolved. But glimmers of the kind of person Harvey had been remained. The clerk behind the counter found him charming and amusing. She kept commenting on how much he looked like the comedian Steve Martin. When he hesitated during the test, unsure what the correct answer was, instead of letting him fail, the clerk gave him prompts for the correct answer. To sympathetic outsiders like her, nothing seemed dramatically amiss because Harvey did not look sick. I knew better.

In fact, one of my main purposes in visiting the neurologist was to enlist outside support for my belief that Harvey shouldn't drive anymore. Harvey had recently offered a ride home to a colleague who lived in the neighborhood. Simple directions became a maze of missed turns that they both joked off as being too preoccupied in their conversation. Harvey's admission that his reaction time behind the wheel seemed slow signaled like a caution light that time was up trying to honor his independence. Someone could get seriously hurt.

After the unsuccessful meeting with the neurologist, I decided to take action. I slipped into the garage one night and pulled the plugs on what I thought were the lines to the battery and circuitry to permanently cripple his car. For the next five years, I told Harvey that his car was in the shop getting repaired. It was an easy fib to maintain. Even then, Harvey didn't have the presence of mind to check the garage himself where the car remained.

The morning of the big lecture, he didn't even ask to drive. He slid into the passenger seat and waited in stony silence for me to take charge. The drive to the hotel was short. Harvey clutched his slide decks on his lap, afraid to let them out of his sight after briefly failing to locate them that morning. I was reluctant to just drop him off at the entrance of the hotel for fear that he might get lost. Fortunately I spotted a member of his staff and commandeered help for Harvey with his briefcase and slide decks. We arranged a place to meet afterward. I parked the car and slipped into the back of the ballroom, standing where he would not see me.

In every Alzheimer's case, there is invariably a public episode that drives home the harsh reality and makes denial no longer an option professionally. That scenario is true for every public figure and celebrity who has ever been forced to own up to the disease. We applaud them as courageous, but they had no choice.

For me and for his increasingly concerned colleagues at work, Harvey's speech that day was such an episode. It was painful watching this brilliant man, renowned for his expertise in blood cancers, fumbling with his papers. Though he held the typed speech in front of him, he lost his place less than halfway through and never recovered. There were awkward pauses while he tried to retrace the steps of his argument. I heard attendees shifting in their seats, rustling papers, craning their necks to see him and try to understand what was going on. At one point, an uncomfortable rumble of laughter, a kind of snickering, seemed to wave across the ballroom. I wanted to stand up and shout to this room full of doctors with fancy titles and prestigious sinecures, supposedly trained in spotting the clinical symptoms of a disease, "Can't you see this man is sick and needs help?" But I was so afraid of embarrassing Harvey even more that I stood there silently, waiting for it to be over. Finally, one of the organizers gently led him to his seat. He never finished the speech.

On the drive back from the hotel, I felt bitter and angry about what had just happened. When we walked into the house, the first thing I noticed on the table in the front hallway was a bill from the neurologist who had found nothing wrong with Harvey. I crumpled the bill into a wad and threw it in the trash. I refused to pay.

Despite my regular talks with Henry Masur, I did not know that a few of Harvey's colleagues had started talking to the administration-level managers about easing him out of his job. At the very least, they insisted, management needed to get Harvey thoroughly examined. In the lab that Harvey was nominally running, the day-to-day responsibilities fell to his two deputies. It was hard for them to do their own work and Harvey's too. At the suggestion of these colleagues, Harvey's boss attended the speech. He was shocked by Harvey's demeanor and performance.

The next morning, Harvey's boss called him into the office and told him that under no circumstances was he allowed to see patients. He needed a clean bill of health and the last report didn't count. Harvey promised to limit his work to the lab. His two deputies were also called to the front office and assigned to keep an eye on him. But right after Harvey agreed to the new arrangement, he seemed to forget it. It was an almost impossible task to keep Harvey in the lab and away from the wards.

Harvey wasn't responsible only for himself and the patients. There were fellows and graduate students whose career advancement depended on Harvey. They needed his help to supervise their research and shepherd their papers through the review process and into publication in prestigious journals. They wanted him to mentor them. All of this he was now unable to do. Morale in the lab started to flag.

Less than two weeks after Harvey's final speech, he was supposed to fly to London for a meeting of the FAB—for French, American, and British—leukemia classification committee. Harvey had been invited to join years back, and it was one of the highlights of his career. There was one other American on the committee; everyone else was based in Europe. This meant

regular trips to Paris, his favorite city, and to London, a city
he also had gotten to know very well.

Harvey wanted to attend the meeting in London, but after
the confusion he had exhibited during the speech, I was terribly concerned. He rejected my offer to come with him. The
situation had the makings of a disaster.

This was the most challenging point in his illness, when
Harvey stood on the border between who he had always been
and what would characterize the rest of his life. For a while, he
had been able to keep one foot on each side. There were days
when he was still his old self, with flashes of the intelligent and
funny Harvey. He would make a joke or refer to something that
happened in the news. He could make conversation, and he had
strong opinions about what he wanted to do. But then, without
warning, his eyes would glaze over and he would get a distant,
vacant expression. He seemed to be looking off in the distance,
perhaps at the fate that awaited him. I worried that he would
not be able to keep himself together for the long overseas flight.
Harvey still maintained the demeanor of a high-functioning
man. If he fell apart, who would be there to help him?

I had lost whatever influence I once had over him. He was
far enough into the early stages of mild cognitive impairment
to be obstinate and unwilling to listen to reason. My tears and
pleading that he should stay home fell on deaf ears. The visit
to the neurologist who had told Harvey he was fine turned out
to be the one episode he did not forget. Now I had lost my

standing as his defender. Harvey treated me as his enemy; someone he could not trust. By this point, we were the only ones
living at home. There were no allies to help me dissuade him
from leaving for London.

A dementing mind sees only its own reality.

The morning of the flight, he frenetically packed his bags.
The process took two hours because he kept unpacking and
repacking, yet he still managed to forget to take his grooming
necessities, which he left scattered on the bathroom counter.
Pants and shirts were strewn all over the bed. I offered to help,
but he slammed the door. I stood quietly outside in the foyer
in case he called for me. The next thing I knew, a cab was
honking at the front door. I confronted Harvey in the doorway, saying that if he was leaving, he should first check to
make sure he had his passport, his plane reservation, a ziplock
bag of pounds and francs that he carried on every trip, and his
itinerary. Everything was there. Rote memory was still suffi-
ciently intact for him to give me a good-bye kiss. I reminded
him to call me when he landed.

He managed to get himself on the plane, and the hosts of
the committee meeting arranged for a driver to pick him up at
the airport. They were all staying together in a small boarding
house in Kensington, a place they had stayed during other
meetings in London. The familiarity of the place seemed to ease
Harvey's agitation, at least at first. But soon after he arrived,
things started to go wrong.

During the first day of the meeting, when all the scientists were staring at the slides in their microscopes and taking notes, his friends started to notice that Harvey wasn't participating. He would press his eyes against the microscope, but he didn't seem to see anything. His notebook lay untouched beside the microscope. When he did finally make a note, it was gibberish. One of his closest colleagues asked him if he was feeling okay, and he admitted that he was not. He asked to go back to the hotel. For the remaining two days of the conference, he barely left his room. The meeting fell apart. Instead of debating the leukemia slides, the scientists spent the entire meeting debating Harvey. What was wrong with him? How could they help him? How would he be able to get home?

At one point, Harvey announced to the scientists that he wanted to tell them something important at lunch, but when they got to the restaurant and looked expectantly at Harvey to make his announcement, he appeared to have forgotten he had ever said anything. Instead, he talked on and on about that raven-blue car he had bought during his sabbatical in Paris. He grew agitated as he told his colleagues that he needed to fly there right away, that he had parked his car in a garage, and he needed to retrieve it and find a more secure location.

The other scientists tried over and over to persuade him to go straight back to the United States. They told him he needed to see a doctor, that he was not well enough to travel to Paris. But he insisted that he be driven to the airport to catch a flight to France, and there didn't seem to be any way to force him to come home. They arranged for a colleague they knew to meet him at the airport and take him into town, but when he arrived in Paris, he caught a taxi to a hotel.

I was frantic. I had known from the start that this trip was too much for him; the stress of traveling abroad and having to make so many decisions would ultimately leave him unable to function. But I was stymied by the same obstacles that had made it impossible to keep him from going to London or for his colleagues to prevent him going to France. There was no diagnosis. He insisted on taking care of himself and making his own decisions, even though his decisions no longer made sense. Yet he was still able to rise to the occasion and fool those who didn't know him well—a taxi driver who didn't realize the extent of his disorientation or the flight attendants on Air France, who never asked if he needed help.

In Paris, Harvey eluded his colleagues for two days. Even now, I am not sure where he went. I later learned that he persuaded a bank teller to let him close out his personal account; the money was never recovered. He kept telling people he wanted to drive his car but could never locate the keys.

I kept calling his colleagues in Paris, asking them to try to help locate him and to see if anyone traveling back to the United States might be persuaded to assist him. I was terrified by the thought of his getting rerouted and lost. I was also afraid to fly to Paris to retrieve him myself, fearing he might escape me too. Colleagues eventually tracked him down, but his return ticket was changed five times. Harvey refused to believe that he needed to go home right away.

While I continued to try to arrange Harvey's flight back, I made contact with a female colleague who had been at the London meeting. It was summertime, and we sat outside a hotel in Bethesda. She told me she was the only scientist that Harvey had allowed to care for him after he locked himself in his room. He had confided that he felt scared and confused.

Years later, when colleagues at the London meeting recalled the events, they remembered the rapport Harvey had with this scientist. They speculated that perhaps Harvey connected with her because it was her first time attending the meeting. He did not feel as embarrassed with her because she had never known him as he was, and therefore could not judge how much he had changed. I could not help but note that she was very attractive and had also been the only woman at the London meeting. The intimacy of the episodes she described made me wonder in a brief, jealous moment if they were somehow linked romantically. But then the reality of Harvey's condition sank in. This was not romantic at all; she was genuinely distraught to see a colleague unravel. I frantically wrote down the details she described and shared my frustration that similar symptoms in the past had still not resulted in a diagnosis. I took her card and asked if Harvey's next round of doctors might

contact her directly. Perhaps if they heard the story from another doctor, they might believe that Harvey was on a slow,
but irreversible course of cognitive decline.

I finally succeeded in arranging for a Paris research colleague
en route to Los Angeles to accompany Harvey to Charles de Gaulle
Airport, help him navigate through customs, and make certain
he was on the right flight home. Harvey was supposed to arrive
in Dulles around 2:40 P.M. Sunday. Arriving at the airport three
hours early, I gained the sympathy of an airport police officer
who had suffered head trauma and short-term memory loss. He
escorted me in to explain the circumstances to the immigration
officials. When I pointed out my husband in the crowd, Harvey
didn't look like someone who was impaired or even confused.
He was well dressed, his appearance neat. I felt the sympathy
my story had garnered starting to slip away. I wondered if they
suspected that I concocted the story to earn special treatment.
Once back, Harvey was like a recalcitrant little boy who knows
he has done something mischievous but doesn't realize for a
moment that he could have been seriously harmed.

The trip to London, coming so close on the heels of his
breakdown during the lecture to the doctors, was the final straw
for me. I knew that we had to get Harvey a real diagnosis.
Even though it was Sunday, I drove Harvey directly from the
airport to the office of a physician and close personal friend to
run a battery of tests and persuade Harvey that he had to go to
the hospital for further brain scans.

The next day we went to see a brain trauma expert at the
National Naval Medical Center right outside of Washington,
D.C. There, my husband, Captain Harvey R. Gralnick could
have his medical records from his thirty-one years in the public health service matched with his most recent X-rays. I was
desperate to identify why Harvey today was not the man I
married. Some may wonder why I didn't do this at the very
beginning. The answer: any results from these tests would immediately go into his work record and be reported to his superiors. Why put his career in jeopardy if it was something that
could be diagnosed without fanfare and treated elsewhere?

I remember the moment when I first heard the words I had
been chasing for the past two and a half years. I was leaning
against a filing cabinet, directly behind Harvey and halfway
out the door of a cramped office, while he sat bewildered across
the table from the doctor, whose shoulders now slumped as the
bearer of onerous news: "A comparative of brain scans done
after his 1985 car accident almost a decade before shows actual
shrinkage as well as plaques and tangles in the hippocampus
region of the brain. His PET scan offers us a 65 percent certainty that Dr. Gralnick's condition presents as a form of dementia. It may even be Alzheimer's. It is atypical in a person
of his age, education, and level of physical fitness. Have you
ever heard of it?"

The word *Alzheimer's* hung in the air. Harvey said nothing.

His mind had already become a sieve in such technical conversations. I had never heard of the disease, and no doctor had ever mentioned it. Could he be mistaken? What were our options? How fast does the disease progress? What's in store for us? Wouldn't it be prudent to get a second opinion, since my husband presents differently each time he is seen and there is no medical consensus?

Just then the doctor's pager went off, and he stood apologetically to dismiss us, saying there was an emergency and he was on call. But before he left, his final words set me on the next course of action: "Unfortunately, if it is Alzheimer's, there is no cure for this fatal neurodegenerative illness—and only four drugs available to treat symptoms. Under regulations I am required to report my findings, though not definitive, immediately to his agency head at the NIH."

The doctor disappeared into a nearby doctors-only elevator. Harvey and I were left behind to deal with the consequences and figure out what to do next. Harvey's face was a blank. It wasn't even clear he had heard or understood the doctor's diagnosis. He looked up at me and said, "Isn't it time for lunch?"

I knew I had to move fast. His X-rays were still on the desk as was the doctor's report. I slipped both sets of medical records into my bag and left a brief note on the doctor's desk. "Will return tomorrow. Need to copy for our records and second opinion."

At work, the question about what to do about Harvey had already been set in motion. No one was willing to wait for a formal diagnosis. The news about Harvey's breakdown in London quickly got back to his colleagues at the NIH. People were shocked and worried. By then, everyone understood that, whatever Harvey had, it was progressing and unlikely to get any better. This was the beginning of the end of his career, and I knew I had to somehow find a way for him to leave and preserve his legacy. I drove him to work while I searched for a solution, but things took on a momentum of their own.

One day, a prominent cancer researcher who had trained with Harvey came to the NIH to speak with a group of young fellows. He asked during his visit to see Harvey. One of the doctors there warned the visitor that he might find Harvey changed, that he was struggling with a medical issue. When Harvey's colleague saw him, Harvey seemed lucid. "They told me you have Alzheimer's," said the doctor. His colleague's words came as a total surprise. There had yet been no official diagnosis of his medical problem. Harvey came home angry, upset, and frightened. I complained to human resources that no one should be discussing Harvey's medical issues or making their own diagnoses.

Then I got a devastating phone call. Several women in Harvey's lab had filed sexual harassment claims against him, saying he used inappropriate language and they felt uncomfortable working with him. I went in with our lawyer and

Harvey to discuss what to do next. I felt angry and bitter during the entire conversation. Throughout his career, Harvey always promoted women scientists. His deputy was a woman, and he supported women's careers. Now I felt that they were looking for a way to force Harvey out. I could never be entirely sure whether he had said the things the women claimed he did.

One of the devastating effects of the illness is that it lowers people's inhibitions. They often say and do socially inappropriate things as incipent dementia takes hold. Still, some of the claims seemed contrived. If the charges stuck, it would make Harvey ineligible for his pension and leave a tarnished footnote that overshadowed his remarkable career.

It took less than a day to resolve his case. Harvey would retire with disability but would no longer be permitted on the NIH campus, effective immediately. For over thirty years, this place had been the center of Harvey's daily existence. He knew every corner of the campus, and now he was no longer welcome there. We drove home in silence. Only I fully understood that this was the end.

"And what will be his legacy?" I wondered in the days and weeks and months that followed. From time to time, there was a call from a former colleague inquiring about Harvey's health. But Harvey was too distracted to make conversation, and I barely knew the people he had seen every day for decades. Most conversations tapered off into awkward silence. We had a few visitors at the beginning, but this too was excruciating to watch. He had trouble remembering them by name, and they certainly were unable to recognize the person he had sadly become. In the end, even these few visitors stopped coming by. It was just the two of us in the house, but I realized I was alone.

THREE

TWO UNCERTAIN WORLDS

The first Monday morning after Harvey had been banned from the NIH campus, he paced aimlessly around our home like a man under house arrest. He was dressed for work, but he had nowhere to go.

Harvey had only selective recall of what had happened at the fateful meeting at the NIH. Sadly, I reminded him that he had no options right now, but to work from home. "Love, let's think of it as a sabbatical until we find out what's wrong." That's all I could say as I cleared the dining room table to arrange an office on the first floor. But he had latched onto the notion that I was the one responsible for his predicament. That made me the prime target for his unpredictable and unprovoked rage.

I was already late for work but afraid to leave him alone. Our housekeeper, Anna, had been with the family for years.

Harvey's paranoia was growing and this was no time to bring in a stranger, so I had hired Anna's daughter, Olga, who worked as a nursing aide in a Quaker-run assisted living facility, to be his part-time companion.

I knew we were fortunate to be able to bring in help, but even then, I was already worried about our finances. Harvey had been forced into early retirement, and his disability pension was $59,000 a year. He had no long-term care insurance. My career was also in transition. After eighteen years as a syndicated business show host and news anchor, my new assignment was to lead the re-launch of the U.S. Chamber Foundation. Under the circumstances, I wasn't sure how long I could keep working.

Even with hired backup, the act of leaving the house for work was an arduous task. Harvey's doctor prescribed a sedative to be given if he got too agitated. As a precaution that morning, I slipped half a tablet in with his vitamins. Harvey spit them back at me. I gave up trying, anxious to deflect any confrontation. Then I called his lawyer who was prepared to recap with Harvey why he could not go back to NIH. We both hoped that hearing the familiar voice of a trusted friend might calm and defuse his misplaced anger. I reminded Olga not to let Harvey out of her sight as I slipped out the front door and headed off to work.

That day I had an important meeting, but halfway downtown, I got a frantic call from Olga. Harvey had pushed her aside when she tried to block his exit at the front door. He was already a good distance up the street and headed for Cedar Lane, a rigorous three-mile trek to the NIH. A long-distance runner, Harvey could move fast, but he was carrying two heavy briefcases and wearing slip-on loafers. I knew because I had helped him dress before I left for work. I turned the car around, backtracking to cut him off before he came to any harm.

A return trip that should have taken fifteen minutes took only ten, as I raced through side streets and cut through alleys, like a flashback to my adrenaline-driven reporter days when I raced to be first on a crime scene. Turning off Wisconsin Avenue past the NIH complex onto Cedar Lane with no Harvey in sight, I made a U-turn and headed in the direction of the Clinical Center, where Harvey used to see his patients. The route was devoid of pedestrians. What about Rock Creek Park, which intersected Cedar and where we ran on weekends? I had just driven under the overpass before Beach Drive when I noticed in the distance a solitary figure propped awkwardly against a tree. As I approached, I saw it was Harvey. Next to him stood like sentinels the two briefcases filled with research he would never finish.

I pulled onto the gravel strip and jumped out of the car. "Hi, love," I said to him, trying to feign a nonchalance I did not feel. "Need a ride home?" Harvey did not look surprised to see me there in the middle of the park. He merely looked up and said he had spent the morning at the NIH Library doing research and thought he would walk home for lunch. It was only 10:30, and I knew that he had never made it there, but I said nothing. He did not inquire why I wasn't at work.

We sat together for a few minutes while I debated how to cajole him to come home with me. Fortunately, Harvey began to get hungry since he had refused breakfast. I reached out to pick up one of his briefcases but the anger in his eyes made me recoil. I felt stung by his unspoken admonition that he did not need my help. He asked about his car again and why he couldn't drive himself to the office. I told him it was in the shop so we'd have to commute together, but the only place he was going that day was home. Even after we arrived back at the house, I remained terribly shaken by the turn of events. I called work and canceled the rest of my meetings for the day.

With Harvey now home all day, I tried hard to keep things as normal as possible. It was maddening, but I just quietly played along as if it were the first time I had heard, "When can I go back to work?" "Where's my car?" "How come you are in my house?" "Do I know you?"

The most pressing issue was figuring out what was going wrong with Harvey. I wasn't sure how to explain my current home situation at work. Under new leadership, the broadcasting division had been decimated, our ranks stripped away, the studio emptied, and jobs reassigned. Any request for time off would be viewed critically. There was no way to manage Harvey at home without devising a better plan. My accrued vacation time combined with sick leave would give me six weeks to try to pin down a diagnosis. I needed to be careful not to jeopardize my position at work. Right now, my job was our sole source of income.

At first, I tried to engage Harvey in the quest for information about his symptoms, but that once-brilliant mind could no longer remember the most basic tasks. He began needing prompts on how to button his shirt and reminders to bathe and to brush his teeth. There were days when he engaged in endless repetition and others when he said nothing at all. It was hard to decide which I disliked more. But if you asked him directly how he was, he answered that he was fine.

We only had a short time before my leave would end, so I pressed to have Harvey seen by a prominent neurologist and physician at Johns Hopkins. The wait was six months. I wrote a letter to the then president, citing my husband's contributions in the research community and requesting an urgent second opinion. Perhaps Johns Hopkins, one of the leading research hospitals, could help me solve the mystery of Harvey's symptoms.

Two weeks later, armed with his test results, MRI scan, and my typed observations, we entered the outpatient assessment center in Baltimore. To protect Harvey's privacy, instead of using his real name, I wrote in the name of his favorite '82 Bordeaux, a reminder of better days. For the next week he was known as Peter Petrus.

Still, even at this top-ranked medical institution, they did not immediately suspect Alzheimer's disease, even after reviewing the diagnosis and charts from the Bethesda Naval Center. Back then, formal diagnosis for Alzheimer's came only with autopsy. It would be a drawn-out process of elimination.

On one trip to Hopkins, we were directed to the office of Dr. Peter Rabins, whose book, *The 36-Hour Day*, had become the bible for Alzheimer's caregivers. Dr. Rabins interviewed us separately and then together. It was the first time I felt a clinician listened to me; the first time one had asked how I was holding up. Rabins sent Harvey for further psychological tests—more endless hours in monochromatic waiting rooms and exam rooms that felt like holding pens for the anxious families.

Although Rabins didn't use the word *Alzheimer's*, when he wrote out a prescription, it was for an antidepressant and Aricept, one of only four drugs available to temporarily moderate the symptoms of dementia. Despite the mounting signs, the doctors still didn't feel they could conclusively diagnose Alzheimer's disease. Harvey's medical condition remained undiagnosed, debated, and unresolved for the next two years.

Between doctor visits, I spent hours trying to put Harvey's papers in order. Harvey had always been a very private person. I searched to no avail for some kind of advance directive so I could execute his last wishes. It had been on our to-do list after we gave each other power of attorney in the event of illness early in our marriage. I also uncovered evidence that Harvey had been having issues since before I had even first suspected. I found three years of signed tax returns that had never been filed stuffed under a dusty pile of research papers on the credenza behind his desk. There were also unfiled patent papers for monoclonal antibodies, research papers left half finished, unpaid parking tickets, an unused certificate for a weekend racing school that we had given him one Father's Day, boxes of old cancer slides, and safe deposit keys that opened doors I knew not where.

Why hadn't I pushed him harder to share important documents and keep information up to date? I turned my anger inward; there was nowhere else to direct it. I had so wanted to believe Harvey when he said that he wanted to take care of me. I was trusting, and it was now coming back to haunt me. How could I have missed his lack of concern, especially about matters that pertained to both of us?

In the evenings, between Harvey's waking hours and the nightmares that made it impossible for him to sleep through the night, I tried to read up on diseases of the brain, searching for ways to try to preserve his motor function. I closely tracked Harvey's behaviors, sleep patterns, and outbursts, looking for a pattern or a clue—something that might offer me a way to help him.

I knew that once I went back to work, it would be harder to find time for the kinds of exercises the books discussed:

stretching and calisthenics to strengthen gait and eye-hand coordination, verbal games involving repetition of phrases and words in a desperate effort to salvage language and skill sets that he was already losing. I started to wonder, "My God, what if he forgets my name?"

My combined leave and vacation time ran out with no diagnosis to show for it. Now I had to go back to work caught between two uncertain worlds and distracted daily by Harvey's growing dependence and unpredictability. By then, Olga and I had devised a routine. She distracted Harvey when I left for the office. I coached her to pretend to be his research assistant, and told her that she could drive him anywhere he wanted to go except for the NIH campus.

During the day at work, I made sure that Harvey and I spoke every hour and sometimes more than once. He needed me to reassure him that I would be home shortly. The frequent and insistent calls were distracting. Every time I sat down to work on a project or concentrate on some task, the phone would ring, a jarring reminder that even here there was no escape from what was happening at home. I switched my hours so I could get home earlier, arriving at work at 7:00 A.M. and leaving at 4:00 P.M., then spending the remainder of the day caring for Harvey. I worked hard to hide my exhaustion, giving myself an extra twenty minutes to meticulously apply makeup—my mask to the world.

Once home, I walked with Harvey for up to six miles to

help alleviate the confusion known as sundowning, when patients with memory issues are most likely to become agitated. I drove him almost every day to the tennis courts near our house. Hoping to help him maintain eye-hand coordination, we hit the ball back and forth in a monotonous rhythm. Still physically agile enough to get to the ball, we would volley, only stopping when Harvey tired or he couldn't focus.

At night, we washed up together in a shower built for two, which we had installed thinking about romance but appreciated now for its practicality. I locked the door to our bedroom, leaving the light on so he could see we were safe, but he still had trouble sleeping, and that meant I was up too—cajoling, comforting, and cradling him when he said he saw snakes crawling on the walls or heard strange voices. His medications were adjusted, but the anxieties remained. I tried ruses to assure him we were safe—screaming at the moonlight that cast shadows through the shades, catching the illusive creatures of the night in pillowcases that I had previously filled with toy rubber vermin—all to persuade Harvey that he could go back to sleep. In this way, night and day often ran together. Soon, weeks and then months slipped by without me noticing. I felt like I lived in a perpetual haze.

I remember him lying in our bed one night early on and furtively staring at me. Then he challenged me on why I was in his bedroom. I quickly pulled a dictating recorder out of my side table, used for sleepless nights when my mind wouldn't turn off, to record the conversation. He didn't recognize me as his wife even when I showed him photos of us together. But it was also the first and last time he ever acknowledged my sacrifice. "If you are in fact my wife," he said, "then what's happening is very unfair to you." I was hoping for more guidance.

What should I do? Divorce him? I loved him and felt committed to our promise to care for one another in either good or bad times.

Put him away in a facility and get on with my life? The regulations back then allowed nursing homes to advertise dementia units without any specific training for their workers, specialized activities, or safety measures in place. Harvey deserved better.

Send him to live with his son in California? Their relationship worked because they were apart except for an occasional phone call, and I quickly dismissed the idea.

Assist him to end it all because without his intellect he was no longer himself? This felt immoral to me and I knew it was something I could never do. For someone like Harvey, hanging around wasted and dependent would be more abhorrent than death. When he was cogent, before the disease took hold of his mind, he had said those exact words but left no written directives.

Harvey's denial about his own descent into disease would be his undoing and my own.

Trips outside the house, even for minor errands or grocery shopping, were fraught with unexpected complications. Harvey's social filters were unraveling and, along with them, his inhibitions and sense of appropriateness. If he had to urinate, this once distinguished man picked the nearest bush, a stack of newspapers at the pharmacy, or the wheel of the car next to ours in the shopping mall. I couldn't easily interrupt him, so I did my best to block the view or remind him to use the bathroom before we walked out the door. I always carried a fresh change of clothes for him. Excursions became more and more limited. Even at home, I sometimes unexpectedly found urine in waste cans, drawers, and as irrigation for houseplants.

As much as possible, I still tried to take Harvey out, hoping that seeing friends might stimulate his fading memory. I exhausted myself bathing, shaving, and dressing him, and then hurriedly dressed myself for the occasional evening out. If we kept moving at a cocktail party, I figured no one would suspect the truth. But by the end of those evenings, I often wondered if the effort and dissembling was worth it. Harvey couldn't tell me where we'd just been or whom we'd seen, even if they were our close friends.

Most people have a bucket list of things to do before they die; mine is a "never again" list. On work assignments that required a night away from home, I had no choice but to take him with me. One particular report was on board a cruise ship docked in Fort Lauderdale. There was no live news feed, so I thought I could manage him. On a docked ship, I figured there were only so many places for Harvey to get lost. I purchased an identification tag and bracelet at the mall and put them on him, but Harvey had never liked wearing anything but a watch, so I was afraid he would take it off. As an additional precaution, I sewed name tags in his clothing, as you would for a child headed for camp. I even taped a strip inside both shoes with information on how to contact me if he got lost.

I hired someone to watch him while I filmed, but almost immediately, Harvey slipped away. Fearing that something bad might have happened, I told the camera crew to shoot the scene without me while I frantically searched the ship. Harvey eventually was discovered at the bar drinking wine and comparing notes with the ship's sommelier. He had already downed several glasses, so I hurried him back to the stateroom, where he promptly passed out. I called the crew and told them to wrap. I grabbed a pillow off the bed and slept on the floor, propped against the door to make certain Harvey didn't disappear again. We disembarked early the next morning.

*As the months wore on, things got worse. Whatever mind-*ravaging illness he had, it now turned him unpredictably violent. I was instructed by doctors to be cautious and call 911 if he got too violent. Harvey was six foot two and 185 pounds; I was fearful all the time.

The biggest problem was that it was almost impossible to anticipate an outburst. He often came up to me from behind, catching me unaware as I cooked dinner or was doing some household chore. I never knew if he was going to try to hug me or choke me. When I noticed that he seemed agitated, I tried to keep a safe distance. I would quietly leave the room and wait a few moments, then walk back in with a "Hi love, anything you need?" or "You asked me to find your keys and here they are," hoping that his anger would have subsided or he would have forgotten what was upsetting him. In a fit of desperation, I installed oversized concave mirrors on the walls between the kitchen and family room, our bedroom, bathroom, and adjoining home office. The mirrors were designed to let me see around blind corners, allowing me to monitor him from another room. If he seemed angry or agitated, I had a few moments to decide whether to confront him.

This was the bleakest period yet. I felt trapped in my own home. Then my world opened up a bit with the birth of my first grandchild, a precious baby girl named Hope. She was doll-like, less than six pounds with perfect little features. I watched Jason through the glass window, hovering over her in intensive care. It was a disquieting scene because it reminded me how helpless and how dependent we are on doctors for answers. All the while, Harvey was regressing. Even though I have a photo of the two of us holding Hope in the hospital room, Harvey never knew Hope or any of his five grandchildren. I quickly realized it was too difficult to take Harvey with me when I wanted to see Hope, Eli, and Benjamin. I paid a nurse to stay extra hours while I drove to my son's house to help care for and play with my grandchildren. It lifted my spirits to see how each of them responded to me as their "Nana." The unconditional love and energy I poured into them came back in very direct and honest ways. They were my antidepressant of choice; the only joy in my life, filling me with hope where there was none.

At home with Harvey, I worked harder and harder, but the person I loved was disappearing bit by bit mentally and physically right before my eyes.

At our visit to Hopkins, Dr. Rabins had warned me that over time, as Harvey's symptoms got worse, the efficacy of the medication he had prescribed would likely diminish. At some point, the dosage levels might need to be adjusted. It didn't take long before this happened, but I kept quietly trying to manage the situation alone through phone consults. The doctor had already increased the antidepressant when I began having trouble coaxing Harvey to get up in the morning. Even with the increased dose, I often had to wake him by saying, "Dr. Gralnick, your patients are waiting. They need you." Though that seems cruel, it was truly the only way to get his cooperation. By the time he was dressed, he had already forgotten the ruse.

I frantically looked for options to tame his symptoms. I played New Age music at night and used aromatherapy; I pumped up his favorite rock 'n' roll from the 1970s so loud he could hear it anywhere in the house. Nothing seemed to help. There were also signs of physical deterioration. I noticed that Harvey had difficulty negotiating the steps up to the second-floor bedroom. He was fearful and timid, sometimes taking nearly fifteen minutes to mount a flight of stairs. Was it a depth perception issue? Would a new prescription for eyeglasses help? I took him to see the doctor, but the eye exam was inconclusive.

Time weighed heavily for both of us. I checked off each month like a scorecard and test of my own resilience. Another two years passed.

It was clear that Harvey was slowly and progressively getting worse. If anything, his anxieties seemed more pronounced despite the medications. He shadowed me around the house, refusing to leave my side. Sweating profusely, he continuously paced the family room or kitchen. It got harder to stay out of his way. I tried to come up with strategies to protect myself but usually had no time to prepare. Harvey's anger came from someplace out of my reach. It was like a sudden summer storm, his face quickly turning menacing. Often he grabbed my wrist in a crushing grip. Unable to pull free and fearing he might break my arm, I would deliberately move closer to him. I kept my head and chin down so he couldn't get at my throat with his other hand. Then I would hug him with my free arm and say as calmly as the rising fear would allow, "You are a great doctor. You help people, not hurt them. I know you are frustrated, but I am the one who helps you." I kept on talking until something in my conversation or tone distracted him enough to make him loosen his grip.

Other times, if he grabbed both my wrists, effectively pinning me in place, I would break down in tears, hoping to bewilder or confuse him enough that he would let me go and walk out of the room. But I realized we could not go on like this; if the situation continued or deteriorated even further, I could end up getting seriously hurt.

I spoke again with Dr. Rabins who felt it was time for another round of testing. He recommended that Harvey be brought to the hospital and placed under observation to adjust his medication and look for a better diagnosis than dementia. I was reluctant, knowing that Harvey felt safe at home and unsure how he would behave in a strange environment. But at this point, I felt I had no choice. Things were already bad, and there was nothing I could do to comfort him. Harvey's latest symptoms were adding up to a disturbing prognosis. I started to make the necessary arrangements.

I was desperate for a formal diagnosis even as Harvey was oblivious.

I will never forget the morning we checked into Johns Hopkins Hospital on Meyer 6, a lockdown floor reserved for patients with complicated neuropsychological conditions that cannot be managed elsewhere. As we prepared for what was expected to be a short hospital visit, Harvey was more anxious than normal. I dressed him like a gentleman right down to his best cologne, so the nurses would treat him with respect. Even if they didn't know who he was, they would be able to tell that he was someone of stature, even if he now had trouble getting dressed and kept repeating himself.

Hospital check-in wasn't until 12:30 P.M., so we found seats in the cafeteria, but neither of us could eat. We walked around the outdoor garden before going upstairs. Harvey was very quiet and held my hand like a child. I kept talking, reassuring him that we were going to see if we could adjust his medicines so he would feel better.

"Then can I go back to work?" he asked. Even after everything that had happened, Harvey was fixated on recapturing the life he once had. I would have done anything to help him get it back.

"Of course, love, that's why we're here. The doctors will run some tests and soon things will be just the way they were," I told him.

My reassuring words contradicted the sight that greeted us when the elevator door opened. We stepped into a small, beige chamber with a heavy locked metal door and reinforced wired glass windows. The nurses' voices sounded disembodied as they spoke to us through an intercom and buzzed us in. I kept telling myself that Harvey was scheduled for only three to four days of testing and medication adjustment. If it helped him, a few days in this place was worth it.

We were led to a drab double room just down the hall with sad beige walls and a bathroom devoid of sharp instruments to prevent the patients from wounding themselves. I wasn't sure how Harvey would adjust to a stranger in the room, but there were no private singles available. The nurse assured me that no one was scheduled in, so he would be alone.

Harvey was tired from being up so much of the night before, so he lay down on the bed as I quickly unpacked. I had brought along an old radio to keep him company, since Harvey couldn't work a CD player anymore, and turned it to a channel that played his favorite classical music. If he woke up in the middle of the night and was disoriented, I hoped he would hear the music and relate it to the comfort of home.

Just then, a senior resident entered the room and apologized for not shaking my hand. "Spreads germs, you know. Our mission here is to make certain the patients' best interests come first."

The doctor then turned to Harvey, who sat docilely at the edge of the bed. "You've come to the right place," he told Harvey. "No one can figure out what is wrong with you, Dr. Gralnick."

"That's because nothing is wrong with me and I just want to get back to work. Let's get this over quick," retorted Harvey.

Nothing in this hospital felt familiar except that sudden flash of Harvey's flickering personality. For a brief moment, he almost sounded like his old self. I wondered if I should take him home. The only thing that stopped me was the realization that, even if I did, it would only be a matter of time before we had to return.

FOUR

OUT OF REACH

*I*t was 6:00 A.M. the next day. I had promised Harvey that I would be at the hospital when he woke up, even if it was unlikely he would remember.

There was no one at the nursing station when I arrived, and the cleaning crew paid no attention when, against rules, I slipped into Harvey's room. There he was, sitting slumped on the edge of the bed staring strangely past me. His eyes were glazed. His words came out garbled and slurred. It was clear to me that he had been drugged.

What had happened in those twelve hours when I wasn't by his side?

What trouble had he gotten into? Had he assaulted someone? Why hadn't they called me?

My mind raced with questions. I felt panic and guilt rising that I had left him at the hospital. "Love, do you know who I am?" I asked. Hoping to wake him from his stupor, I held out a cup of his favorite espresso roast coffee I had brought from home.

Nothing. He mumbled but said nothing intelligible. I took his face in my hands and looked directly into eyes that appeared not to see me. "I'm Meryl. I'm your wife, and you are safe. Can you say, 'Meryl'?" Again, only garbled and disconnected words came back to me. In the admission meeting, I had requested that I be allowed to stay overnight to ease Harvey's transition to a place away from home. The doctor had refused, saying it was against rules and there were no exceptions.

I helped Harvey back into bed, and then went searching for answers. The attending physician had just left the floor and the head nurse was in conference, so I stationed myself in front of the nursing station, refusing to move. I demanded to see Harvey's chart but was told it was under review and not available. Finally, a nurse stepped out of the morning rounds meeting to deal with me.

"I brought an anxious man into this world-class hospital to be evaluated, and overnight you've turned him into a zombie," I told the nurse. "What happened? I want to see my husband's chart immediately so I can report back to his neurologist and primary care physician." The nurse promised to get a doctor to speak with me after the morning meeting. I left the door to Harvey's room ajar so I could see if he got out of bed and still be front and center when the meeting adjourned. This time, I wasn't going anywhere.

· · ·

"Haldol—it's an old-line antipsychotic we regularly use to manage aggressive behaviors in dementia patients in case they act up. It was given by the night nurse as a precaution," explained the doctor.

The words "in case he acted up" screamed in my head. "Was my husband's behavior in any way aggressive toward the nurse? Did she feel threatened?" I asked suspiciously. Harvey had been given anti-anxiety medicine before to take the edge off his behavior but nothing this powerful, nothing with this kind of adverse reaction.

The doctor took his time reviewing the chart before he answered. "The night nurse must have noticed on the admission form that Dr. Gralnick had a history of management issues and ordered a dose of Haldol every four hours as a pro re nata. He is due for another dose soon."

"Have you seen what it has done to my husband?" I said, struggling to get my emotions under control. "He can't speak intelligibly, stand up straight, or walk without listing to one side. Please check him. I am worried that something has gone terribly wrong."

We went together to Harvey's room. He had not moved from the fetal position I had left him in. The doctor tried to wake him, but Harvey did not respond.

The doctor did not seem overly concerned. "He's most likely just sleeping it off," he told me. He agreed to stop prescribing the Haldol. But he told me to expect that Harvey would need to stay longer than the few days I originally expected. They wanted to try another antipsychotic, called Risperdal, to help regulate Harvey's moods. "You deserve a diagnosis," the doctor told me. Then he left the room to tend to other patients. Harvey and I were alone again.

Harvey was still sleeping, so I went to the family waiting room to call his doctor, whose office was just one floor above us in the hospital. What I learned next shocked me. His neurologist, someone I knew and trusted, was not directly overseeing Harvey's case. Once we were admitted to the locked ward, the senior attending doctors were in charge.

"What about the Haldol?" I asked. "He was treated like a wild man without provocation." The doctor assured me that he would put in a courtesy call and monitor Harvey's case but that he couldn't do more.

When I got back to Harvey's room, Harvey was awake and sitting on the edge of the bed. He still seemed dazed. His look was unknowing as he gazed into the distance. It had been just twelve hours, but Harvey no longer recognized me.

I spent the rest of the day trying to get Harvey to acknowledge my presence. I assured him that he would be home soon. I helped him shower and dress, hoping the familiarity of routine might trigger some recognition. I plied him with liquids, hoping it would help flush out the noxious medicine.

His ability to stand slowly improved, and his footing grew more stable, so we ventured out to walk the halls. We circled around three or four times. Then, as we came around once more on the way back to the room, I heard a man screaming profanities. Suddenly, two muscular orderlies rushed into his room. A nurse, injection in hand, came running right behind them. In less than thirty seconds, the corridor was silent again. The eerie quiet upset me more than the outburst. Had they treated Harvey the same way last night?

Without warning, Harvey suddenly left my side and bolted ahead. He was moving quickly, in an erratic weaving pattern. I ran for a wheelchair parked at the far end of the hall and called for help. An orderly responded and together we managed to get Harvey into the wheelchair and back to his room. That episode was just the start of increasingly erratic behavior. Harvey was not the person I had brought in just twenty-four hours earlier. He would never again be the same.

By the time the doctor who had seen us earlier dropped by, it was already midafternoon. "How are you doing, Dr. Gralnick? You're a lucky man. Your wife is a tiger when it comes to you." I couldn't take my eyes off Harvey, whose only response was garbled and unintelligible.

From the start of Harvey's illness, I had never spoken about Harvey's prognosis in his presence, so I asked to speak with the doctor privately. When we were alone, I told him that

Harvey seemed distressed and unable to communicate. "Given Harvey's discipline as a doctor, I had initially hoped that running a few tests in a hospital setting might tap into some long-term memory and perhaps reassure him. But given the day's events, it was clear this had not been the case." I asked again for permission to stay in Harvey's room overnight to help ease his transition.

"It's not allowed, and there are no special privileges because you are a doctor's wife," the physician told me. Before I could protest, he added, "It's also for your own protection." It might take time before the doctors found the right medicine or combination of medicines to help control Harvey's disturbing behavior, he told me. Other than the dementia, Harvey was still fit and strong and could lash out and hurt me. "The best thing you can do is remain calm and let us do our job," he said.

I had been put off the day before, but now I persisted. I tried to argue that I could be helpful. If I was allowed to come in early in the morning and stay longer at night, I could make sure Harvey didn't get into trouble. It was clear they were short-staffed, and my presence would ease the burden on the nurses. The doctor never relented. I got permission to stay on the floor only during visiting hours.

By the end of the day, with the drug out of his system, Harvey could again say my name. His eyes, though still glassy, seemed to focus when I put something like a meal directly in front of him. But he ate only if I fed or handed him finger food;

utensils were too complex to manage. I helped Harvey through dinner. When visiting hours were over, it was hard to say good bye. "Good night, love. When you wake up in the morning, I will be right here," I promised.

Before I left for home, I talked him through our good bye checklist. I reminded him that I had asked the nurses to leave the light on in his room. I told him that I had left notes on the back of the door and the bathroom mirror with my phone number. I assured him that when he woke up, I would be right there with him. When I left the hospital that night, I wasn't sure how much he understood. Tonight it was not only the numbing cold night air that kept me awake on the forty-five-minute drive home.

By the end of the first week, my presence was an accepted part of the hospital routine. The nursing staff didn't seem to mind that I arrived with them at 6:30 A.M. and was the last visitor out the door at 8:30 P.M., when visiting hours ended. I tried to enlist the nurses as allies. Many mornings, I arrived with coffee and sweets, a treat for them after the long and difficult night shift. I relieved them of their chores by helping Harvey clean up, dress, and eat chunk-size food that I brought from home. I kept him engaged by walking the floors for exercise, letting them turn their attention to other patients. When the nurses took Harvey's vital signs, I reported back to them how he was tolerating the different dosages of drugs that the doctors were trying. Often

I felt that the doctors dismissed not only my observations, but even the nurses' reports. Sometimes the nurses wrote in Harvey's chart that he didn't seem to be responding to a particular drug, but I noticed that the doctors continued to increase the dosage. When there was a serious side effect, they would slowly wean him off the compound and begin another.

As a patient in the locked ward, Harvey was not permitted to leave the floor. Desperate to defuse his anxieties, I took him out to walk the halls. Patient rooms lined the perimeter around the glass-shielded nursing station. At the end of the hall was a large activities room with long tables and rows of chairs pushed up against the walls.

There was a mix of patients. Some suffered from mental illnesses like schizophrenia and bipolar disorder. Others had bulimia or anorexia, depression, or had attempted suicide. Then there were those like Harvey, with memory and behavior disorders in need of a diagnosis.

I soon became a fixture on the floor and often made conversation with family members and some of the patients, many of whom seemed lonely and eager to engage. Without my asking, they watched out for Harvey and volunteered details about how he was managed or, in their opinion, mismanaged by the staff. A young female anorexic with insomnia whispered to me that Harvey roamed the halls all night unsupervised. Almost all the drugs they tested on Harvey had troubling side effects: high fevers, vomiting, unsteady gait, slurred speech. What had started out as a few days in the hospital for observation now stretched into the third week, with no end in sight.

One morning during the third week, I arrived at 6:45 A.M. to find that Harvey was not in his room. It was empty, and I started to panic. What had happened? I spotted a worn burgundy leather couch, typically located in the lounge area, blocking the entrance to a small room on the other side of the hall. Noises emanating from the room sounded familiar. I peeked in and found Harvey, dazed and pacing back and forth, making a small circuit from the far corner of the bed to the sink, as if he were caged. I called his name, but he did not respond. Moving the heavy barricade just enough to squeeze by, I slipped into the cramped quarters, talking gently and trying to calm him. I held out the breakfast I had brought from home, but he lashed out with his fist. The food landed on the floor, splattering everywhere. I kicked what I could under the bed and threw down a towel so Harvey wouldn't slip, then pulled the nurse's cord for help. No answer.

Harvey now headed straight toward me. There was no room to get out of his way. It was clear that he didn't recognize me. The menacing look in his eyes was frightening. Fearing for my safety, I jumped over the back of the couch onto the cushions, escaped into the hall, and headed for the nursing station. I was told that Harvey had suffered an adverse reaction to a higher dose of the latest medication and was out of control.

Short-staffed, the overnight nurse said there was no option but to move him into the barricaded room where they could monitor him at a safe distance.

I felt sick inside and ran to the ladies' room, where I threw up. Splashing cold water on my face, I tried to pull myself together. I went back to the room and stationed myself near the couch so Harvey could hear me. I hoped the sound of my voice might calm him, but he continued to pace. Eventually, exhausted from his all-night exertions, he lay down on the bed and fell asleep.

A few hours later, he awoke. He seemed calmer but still out of reach. He needed to be cleaned up. I guided Harvey down the hall to the double-stall handicapped shower that accommodated wheelchairs, hoping that the wide berth would give me room to maneuver if I needed to get out of his way. I had been helping him with his personal care for years using a combination of strategies. I tried to give him as much autonomy as possible, even if the act of bathing and dressing took four times longer than normal to complete. I never raised my voice, pretending to be calm even when panicked. However, ever since Harvey had been in the hospital, things were different. Harvey reacted violently to all personal assistance with intimate care and toileting.

I reached with the bath sponge to wash Harvey's groin area and suddenly felt his left fist slam into my face. Blood gushed from my mouth as I backed away, realizing that the force of the blow had smashed my front teeth. I began to cry from the shock and pain.

Harvey seemed confused by the sound of crying, but he never unclenched his fist. I pressed the call button, and the nurse and an orderly came running. Between the two of them, they managed to get control of Harvey. They dried him off and dressed him while I iced my mouth. Each day since Harvey fell ill, I felt that I was slowly losing pieces of my husband, but this episode was a turning point. All the strategies that had once calmed him were failing. He didn't seem to respond either to medicine or to my familiar touch. All I saw now was the dark side of his mind. Harvey was locked away not only in the hospital but inside this strange insidious illness. For the first time, he seemed completely out of reach.

*The weeks in the hospital blurred together. The relentless pac-*ing continued at all hours, with Harvey stopping only to sleep. I fed him while he paced an empty activities room. When he passed by, I reached out with food or drink, hoping to distract him or slow him down. It never did. Even bumping into furniture did not seem to slow him down. My only recourse, another made-in-the-moment solution, was to outfit him with the style of shin guards used by lacrosse players.

Sometimes when I arrived, Harvey was turning a corner or approaching down a long corridor. He walked like a man on a mission, but his eyes were empty and dull. It took four orderlies to hold him down for a simple blood draw. Efforts to help him with mundane activities of living turned even more confrontational. His prognosis worsened. No one had any answers.

One morning while showering him, I noticed that the lower part of his left leg was swollen and inflamed. I reported my observations, first to the nurse and then to the doctor, who ignored me until they ran some tests. Harvey had the beginning of a serious deep vein thrombosis—a blood clot.

The doctor immediately prescribed the blood-thinning agent Coumadin and told me Harvey would have to go on immediate bed rest. Harvey could not stop pacing and he was oblivious to explanations of why he needed to lie down. Four strong male orderlies entered his room. Two held him down while the other two bound his hands and feet with thick leather restraint cuffs. Harvey writhed in pain and cursed angrily. Sweat spewed from every pore of his tormented face. A nurse shot him with a strong sedative, but it did not immediately work. His body contorted and writhed with an adrenaline surge. The doctor ordered me to leave the room, but I refused.

"Let my husband loose," I yelled. "If walking is his way out of this nightmare, then let him walk. He would not consider this living anyway." Harvey was now drenched in sweat and exhausted from his struggles. I felt exhausted too—from Harvey's suffering and the fruitless search for answers.

This sickening scene haunted me and colored every decision I would ever make about his care. Never again would

Harvey be left in a situation where he might be restrained against his will or overmedicated.

Right now I wanted to go home and take Harvey with me.

*With this latest incident, the doctors were running out of op-*tions. They had already run through most of the antipsychotic and psychotropic drugs in their arsenal. None of the drugs seemed to make a difference. Harvey retreated further. He could no longer participate in the battery of cognitive evaluations that the doctors once gave him. After over two and a half months in the hospital, it was time to release him with their best attempt at a formal diagnosis.

A meeting was called for Friday. Jason and I attended. Harvey was in the room too but did not seem to understand anything the doctors and social workers said as they gave their reports. Harvey's incessant pacing continued throughout the conversation.

"I want you to know we have done our best with a very challenging case," the doctor said. He had trouble looking directly at me. "Your husband has presented atypically all along."

Harvey's file lay open on the table, but my eyes were too filled with tears to read the words. The doctor continued, reading aloud from his notes. "Our conclusive findings are that Dr. Harvey Gralnick, age fifty-eight, suffers from early-onset Alzheimer's disease with a behavior disorder."

Finally a diagnosis, even if they seemed to have reached the conclusion by ruling out every other possibility. Before I had a chance to react, Harvey, still pacing around the room, passed close to me and patted me on the head. It was as if he knew something was very wrong and wanted to comfort me, but had no idea what was happening.

After all this time, hearing the words *Alzheimer's disease* spoken out loud did not shock me. But the doctor's next words did. "It is our view," the doctor concluded, "that your husband is too dangerous to go home." Jason wrapped his arm around me, trying to soften the force of the doctor's edict.

FIVE

A DIFFICULT PATIENT

*E*ach and every one in the room seemed to agree that Harvey could not go home. But no one knew what to do with him.

The social worker had made a list of facilities in our area that might take him. Copper Ridge, an institution affiliated with Hopkins and known for handling difficult cases like Harvey's, was full. In between hours at the hospital with Harvey, I had visited some of the others. Each visit left me depressed about the options. The main entrance and visitor spaces were decorated to mimic "home sweet home" and the nostalgia of a by-gone era, replete with a mixture of cheap chintz, wicker, fake plants, and plastic furniture covers. There was also no pretense about the barren and basic living quarters that lined the communal areas. But the immediate distraction was the sickly smell that greeted me at the entrance. The signal it gave off was a warning flag of neglect. The sweet faux fragrance permeated everything, but could not mask the stench of urine or the odor of unbathed patients parked in wheelchairs along the corridors. Before me were the most vulnerable of patients: if neglected they did not remember and if abused they forgot. I never got used to it.

Almost all these assisted living and total care facilities were designed and managed for the convenience of the staff rather than the patients. If the patient didn't eat quickly enough or became in any way belligerent or difficult to feed, solid food was removed and quickly replaced with a liquid protein drink. Geri chairs were used as restraints (that's now against state laws) and antipsychotics were given at the smallest sign of misbehavior. Doors to the outside gardens were typically locked. Most places were understaffed and they couldn't afford residents wandering off. Someone like Harvey, who could not stop walking, had nowhere to go. At all the places I visited, the 1:7 nursing aide-to-patient staffing ratios met the state requirement, but I was appalled. I knew the endless hours I spent focused on my husband's needs, and there was no institutional equivalent.

There was no pretending that Harvey fit the profile of the older, frail residents boarded at most facilities. Not only did he have a challenging dementia diagnosis, but Harvey was trailed by a medical chart that detailed his every transgression. One agreeable group home, run by a psychiatrist and his wife, cost upward of $100,000 a year. Even at that premium charge, we were rejected and candidly warned placement would be diffi-cult. At several midlevel facilities that only make money if the beds are full, I had to promise to pay for private nursing sup-port to bolster the staff, which more than doubled the monthly charge. Even then, most of the management didn't think they could handle him. I was running out of options.

In that final meeting at Hopkins with the team assigned to our case, the doctor in charge admitted he was uncertain of Harvey's prognosis. "Most early-onset patients don't last too long," he told us. "The trajectory of their dementia is steep, not prolonged."

I already knew that drugs to treat dementia symptoms were not a long-term solution. It was all doctors had right now and we had run through all of them. However there was one point about which he never wavered: I was not to manage Harvey's care alone anymore.

"You have no idea what you are up against," the doctor warned me. "It's dangerous. The care is intense, and you'll just burn out."

Then it was the nurse's turn to manage the details. "Your husband will be discharged in two days. He will be sedated and taken by ambulance to whichever facility will accept him," she said. She handed me a copy of the discharge papers and told me to pick up Harvey's medications at the hospital pharmacy before 5:00 P.M. After two and a half months in the hospital, this was it.

Now I had forty-eight hours to relocate my husband from the locked ward of Meyer 6 to another secure facility. I asked them why Harvey needed to be sedated. "Those are the rules," the doctor replied. But I was weary of their rules designed by lawyers anxious about the hospital's liability and at my uninsured, out-of-pocket expense. I might not be able to take him home, but on this issue at least, things were going to be done my way. "There will be no ambulance and no extra sedation because I am the one who will be left to manage the side effects," I told the doctor. "I will take my chances with Harvey."

With no safety net once we left the hospital, I began calling the very same nursing care facilities I had previously rejected. I set up emergency meetings with three located within a ten-mile radius of home to more easily monitor Harvey's care. There was an opening at Kensington Park, less than five minutes from home. A suite had just been vacated by a couple, so it was larger than the regular rooms. It was located on the turreted corner of the third-floor dementia unit at double the standard rate. I knew that I needed room for Harvey to roam, and this was off the main floor, which should minimize the potential of him getting into trouble or bothering other residents. I asked them to hold the space; I would be there in less than two hours to sign the papers. I kept the appointments with the other places in case we were rejected.

On the way to Kensington Park, I called Olga to see if she

would be willing to come in as a private-duty nurse. I explained the situation: Harvey was no longer the patient she knew. In the months since she had seen him, he had further deteriorated. I was going to need as many private-duty hours as she could give me. I also asked her to recruit a coworker that she thought could manage Harvey. The nursing staff at Kensington Park would be there to double team with care and for backup in an emergency. I would help out too, covering the night shift. But would they even accept Harvey once they saw his discharge papers?

Kensington Park's entrance was framed by white rocking chairs on a porch that ran the entire length of the building, but when I went inside, the familiar repulsive odor greeted me. Pushing past my aversion, I followed the posted signs to the manager's office. Fortunately, the woman who had earlier rejected us was no longer in charge. I cut short the typical admission questions and conceded that Harvey was a difficult patient. I was there to make a deal. I told the manager that I had already hired around-the-clock private-duty nurses and that I would take the double suite to limit my husband's excursions on the main floor. All meals would be managed in his room. He would be permitted on and off the floor only under the strict supervision of his private-duty nurses. Otherwise he was confined to his living quarters with no social interaction whatsoever with patients on the floor. Even with these restrictions, Harvey was admitted on a trial basis. I signed the papers. The smell trailed me out the door.

At home, I ransacked rooms, looking for furniture to bring to the Kensington Park suite later that evening. I packed photos to hang on the walls in the hopes that they might remind Harvey of happier times. I made a mental note to run through escape drills when the nurses and I were together with Harvey. We could not count on the facility's staff arriving in time if he suddenly turned on us. We needed to figure out how to quickly get out of harm's way.

It was now close to 8:00 P.M. Exhausted from the day's events, I could not relax. My mind raced with scenarios I might face when I tried to move Harvey from the hospital. Leaving nothing to chance, I made a run to the supermarket to stock the refrigerator and headed back to the facility to unload groceries and furniture. At 11:00 P.M., I turned off the lights in what would be Harvey's new home.

Harvey was still sleeping when I arrived for the last time at Meyer 6. I was relieved to be getting him out of the hospital but terrified about the day ahead. This time, I brought Jason with me. He knew I might need extra help getting Harvey into the car.

The plan, hatched on the way to the hospital, was for me to sit in the backseat with Harvey on the passenger side so Jason was not in a direct line of attack. I feared that if Harvey got violent and lashed out, Jason was the only one strong enough to control the car and get us safely off the road. I had all Harvey's favorite snacks and an ice chest filled with soda to distract him. It was like a flashback to my preparation for long car trips with my son as a child.

The hospital didn't have any instructions because my discharge plan contradicted their standard protocol. They warned me once more that any change in physical setting might set Harvey off. I signed the final papers. We had until noon to leave.

I tried to keep Harvey's routine that morning as normal as possible. I fed him a light breakfast: food would be my ploy to distract him on the drive. A sympathetic nurse dropped in to say good-bye. As she left, she slipped me a sample pack of Ativan, with the warning, "You may need this on the way home." All that was left was to bathe and dress him. In the shower, I kept repeating, "Love, I'm getting you out of here as fast as I can. It's what you told me you wanted. No more hospitals. I promise." I no longer knew how much of that promise I could keep.

Harvey refused to sit still in the wheelchair so two strong male orderlies escorted us to the car, parked in the fifteen-minute drop-off zone. For five minutes, I tried to cajole him into the backseat. Jason was already in the car and kept calling to Harvey to sit with him. Nothing was working. The cacophony of voices and the noise outside the hospital confused him. He wasn't processing anything and stood paralyzed outside the hospital's doors. So Jason and I exchanged places. I jumped behind the wheel of the driver's seat, pushed the passenger door opened and shouted, "Hi honey, I'm here to pick you up. Let's get out of here and go home." With that, Harvey pulled away from the stunned orderlies and got into the car next to me. Jason shut the door and jumped into the backseat. I locked the doors. We were off. A block away, Jason and I switched seats.

The forty-five-minute ride was harrowing. My greatest fear was that Harvey might panic and try to open the locked car door. In frustration and rage, he might grab the steering wheel, endangering us all. I sat right behind him, gently massaging his neck. I knew it sometimes helped him calm down. When would the Ativan kick in? Would his favorite CDs that we were playing be familiar at all? Outside the hospital walls for the first time in months, did he remember anything about his former life?

Jason successfully navigated downtown Baltimore, riding the timed lights so we didn't have to stop, and pulled onto the 95 South interstate. Just forty-five minutes more to our Connecticut Avenue exit. As soon as it was safe, he maneuvered the car into the right-hand lane, just in case we had to suddenly pull off on the side of the road. I started talking, an upbeat stream of narrative of what we were seeing, in the hopes that some word or image might trigger a memory deep in Harvey's brain. We didn't stop by our home before going to Kensington Park. We pulled off the exit ramp and headed toward Kensington. Instead of turning left to our street, Jason took a right and headed down one block to the park, where Harvey's new residence loomed high on the hill directly in front of us. I had called ahead, and they were expecting us. Olga was already there. She waited with Harvey in the car at the entrance of building 3 while we went in to pick up the keys and drop off his suitcase. Jason felt comfortable enough to take off, teasing me that no one would believe our predicament, and made me promise to call him if needed. Thankful for Jason's help, I was now alone and in charge.

The late afternoon sun felt good on our faces, the air fresh. I longed to set Harvey free for a walk outside before he was confined again indefinitely. A neighborhood sports track was just over the knoll and the grounds. I knew his new quarters would be cramped and thought a long walk might help tire him out. I opened the side door, unbuckled Harvey's seatbelt, and let him go. Off he went up the path toward the track, with Olga and me running to catch up. He was moving so fast I had Olga follow him while I ran the track in the opposite direction, coming toward him in a sandwich formation. When I got closer, I saw him smiling for the first time since his stay in the hospital. Was Harvey laughing too? I was so delighted that I ran toward him with a smile and my arms open wide, but in an instant, his face turned menacing. His smile was gone. He shoved me hard and took off again at a powerful pace. Now I was panicked, worried about how we would control him. I was reluctant to send Olga for help, worried that the nursing home director would conclude that Harvey was too much trouble before we had even walked in the door.

Watching at a safe distance, I noticed that Harvey was fixated on staying on the track. He did not deviate outside the lines and showed no interest in the grass. It struck me that he was replicating his roaming behavior in the ward. On his second quarter mile, he stopped for a moment as if to catch his breath. This time when I moved in to help, he didn't bolt. He looked forlorn and helpless as Olga and I each took one hand. "Haven't you tested me enough today?" I asked him as we led him back. "Come on, let's go—" I was about to say "home," but stopped myself. Any pretense was over.

What should have been a five-minute walk had become a twenty-minute ordeal. We made our way through a side entrance to the building, avoiding the manager's office, and got on an elevator that opened at the third-floor dementia unit, where patients were being brought in for dinner. Unexpectedly, Harvey refused to get off the elevator. With the elevator's alarm bell ringing, Olga ran off to get backup to help us corral him toward his room just seventy-five feet away. Presented with a wheelchair, he refused to sit down, and the nursing aides fearfully backed off. For the next fifteen minutes, we rode the elevator up and down, asking waiting guests to please take the steps. It was obvious we were managing an emergency. Each time we hit the third floor, we made another attempt to coax Harvey off. Finally it worked, but only because he was tired of being confined and wanted to roam.

The door of the suite opened onto a long, narrow corridor that branched off into a small moon-shaped living room and a bedroom just wide enough to accommodate a single bed and a small nightstand. A narrow Pullman kitchen and bathroom were directly off the corridor. It was cramped, but we had made it there safely. Olga helped me set up an air mattress at the foot of Harvey's bed. I wanted to be close but out of reach. The days of sharing a bed were over. I took the night shift and Olga promised to be back at seven the next morning. The night nurse dropped by and reviewed the regulations. It was after midnight before Harvey stopped roaming the room and gave in to staying put in bed. Exhausted, I lay down fully dressed and quietly cried myself to sleep.

Nothing about this new arrangement worked. Our effort at establishing a daily routine around the facility's schedule was met with belligerence from Harvey. Isolated from the other residents and nursing aides, we abandoned their schedule and made up one that revolved around Harvey. The facility's offer of staff support to back up my nurses never materialized. In- stead, the facility's caregivers reported to the head nurse that they were afraid of the aggressive man in suite 309. Side effects of the medication made Harvey pick at the air as if catching imaginary bugs between his fingertips. Without warning, he inappropriately pulled his pants down and up repeatedly. He was unable to tell us when he had to go to the bathroom, so whether inside or out, we carried a plastic urinal and a poncho to shield his behavior from the other patients. In an emergency, I was called first, day or night.

I found myself arguing with management that my team was not getting adequate support. At the same time, they seemed to be trying to build a case that my team was unable to control Harvey.

"This memo is to inform you of the event that occurred on the morning of October 1, 2001, at approximately 8:30 A.M.," read one of a number of memos I started receiving from the facility. *"Dr. Gralnick and his caregiver were in the elevator and I heard his companion say, 'Don't do it, don't do it.' It seemed to me that he was trying to urinate in the elevator. When he exited, I approached him very gently, touched his arm, and asked if I could talk to him. At that point he turned around and shoved me into the elevator. The door started to close, and Dr. Gralnick grabbed me by both of my wrists, in a very violent manner, and exposed himself to me. The caregiver was able to get him off of me, out of the eleva-*

tor on the main floor, and escort him outside the building
for a walk. Dr. Gralnick does not follow instructions. He
scared me to the point where I was shaking when I got to
my office. In my opinion Dr. Gralnick needs a male care-
giver. It is obvious that he could hurt a woman easily if
he becomes violent/aggressive again."

I read these memos in anger and also sadness. I had come
to realize that patient summaries told only half the story. They
were designed to protect the institution if someone complained.
I knew that Harvey's illness made it impossible for him to control his behavior. That said, it seemed improbable that he could
grab someone by both wrists and expose himself at the same
time. Still, I kept silent. If I complained or drew attention to
Harvey's actions, we would be asked to leave.

It was clear that our days there were numbered. Facilities
like Kensington Park did not have the manpower that someone
with dementia needed. Staff was constantly turning over, and
it was hard to make a personal connection with Harvey, who
resisted being fed or washed or changed, even by us.

A week after getting the latest memo, I raised the issue of
a change with my nursing team. How would they feel if we
took Harvey home instead of moving him to another facility,
where similar issues were bound to occur? They greeted the
idea with relief rather than hesitation. The time at Kensington
Park had been hard on them too. We knew that if he exposed

himself again, we would probably be asked to leave. We had tried everything to keep Harvey appropriate and under control. We dressed him in jumpsuits and tried suspenders so he couldn't easily pull his pants up or down, but that usually resulted in us struggling to change him out of soiled clothes. If he exposed himself at home, who would care? We could remove the furniture from the family room, and he could circle the cooking island in the kitchen all day if he wanted.

There were serious issues involved in moving him home. We would be free from the restrictions of Kensington Park, but Harvey hadn't lived at home in six months, and his physical and mental capabilities had deteriorated during his time away. Could he still climb steps to the second-floor master bedroom? If not, how would we bathe him on the first floor? I asked them to weigh the issues and help decide if we needed a strong male nurse on the team. "We need to be prepared for the next round," I told them. "Each move with Harvey is traumatic, so this decision is a big one and we'll make it together." Meanwhile, I quietly began mapping out scenarios for his return home.

Our family was no different than others trying to deal with Alzheimer's disease. Each son had their own distinct way of coping. Mark visited us only twice early in the disease while his father could still communicate; then remained physically absent the next eighteen years. By contrast, Jason wanted to know every detail and did extensive research looking to fix the unfixable. He feared for my personal safety and chastised me for contemplating the idea of bringing Harvey home. Jason knew I hadn't been completely candid with him about Harvey's aggressive behaviors. However, we both agreed that Harvey was unlikely to be allowed to stay for long at the nearby facility. Coming home was the only realistic interim solution until a spot opened up at Copper Ridge. Admission there was taking longer since we required a private room. We were now second on the waiting list. I prepared the paperwork and scheduled a visit for the following week so we could be ready whenever a spot for Harvey opened up.

Back at Kensington Park, Harvey's behavior continued to be problematic. Now I was only permitted to walk the halls with him at night, when the patients were asleep in their rooms. Then, eight weeks after we first arrived, our stay at Kensington Park came to an abrupt end. During a music session, it was reported that Harvey approached a female resident and exposed himself. His caregiver reported that he did not pull out his genitals. It didn't matter. We were told he could not leave his quarters and we had to vacate the premises.

Two days later, we made our way through the empty halls and left before dawn. It was again an ordeal getting Harvey into the car, but there was no dementia guide for our perplexing re-entry home.

We had lived in the same house for close to twenty years, but nothing was familiar to Harvey—not the pictures on the walls, the books on the shelves, or the furniture that we bought to decorate each room. It took three of us thirty minutes to cajole Harvey up two steps to the back door and an hour of trial and error to reach the second-floor landing. Each step was treated like a victory and cheered silently. Once there, we showered him and lead him into the softly lit master bedroom. Noise set him off so it was only my voice that guided his every move. I arranged a pile of decorative pillows into a barricade down the center of our king-size bed. If Harvey saw me sleeping next to him, I risked being attacked as a stranger. The bedside lamp stayed on. Trying to think ahead of his every move was exhausting. I hung a souvenir cowbell from Switzerland on our bedroom doorknob as a precaution in case he tried to sneak out in the middle of the night. We gave him some Ativan mixed in some homemade applesauce and finally he drifted off to sleep.

For the next five days, we lived on the second floor because Harvey had become terrified of the steps. I had been worried he could not walk up the stairs but never planned for him being frightened by the descent. I used those days to reconfigure a small side-room library at the front of the house into a bedroom. I installed Smith and Hawkins iron garden gates instead of a child safety gate to control his movement and keep him away from the steps. I put the sofas and chairs in the family room on heavy rubber bed stilts to make it easier for us to help him to sit down.

How to keep him clean confounded me: a sponge bath was not a solution. Then I remembered the small European bathrooms in the hotels when we traveled—nothing more than a toilet, a small sink with wall tile surrounds, and a drain in the floor so one could also shower. I called a contractor, who showed up the next day with two men to convert the small guest bathroom. The foreman told me the job would take at least two weeks, but after watching me coach Harvey slowly down fifteen stairs from a seated position, one step at a time, they finished in less than a week and presented me a bill for half the original quote. I never thought about how strange we must look to outsiders, but clearly these tough men couldn't believe what they had seen.

Life at home was now limited to the first floor. I priced out the installation of an elevator, but it was the cost of a year's worth of care. The nurses and I worked together, always aware that Harvey could strike out without warning. I brought in an instructor for a session in self-defense and to demonstrate how to unlock Harvey's vice-like grip. My personal survival regimen—a weekly weight-training session with a former pro athlete nicknamed Huggy, who pushed me to my physical max and pumped up my courage.

I devised a daily record so we could track Harvey's moods and behavior; whatever worked we repeated, and then shared techniques. He rarely spoke other than to curse, so we just kept up a cheerful one-way conversation with him while searching for some flicker of recognition or positive response. We prepared his favorite finger foods that he picked up and ate as he wandered the kitchen. Harvey could no longer verbalize his appreciation, so the quirkiest of behaviors became endearing. Any measure of cooperation coaxed out of him scored as a win. But we never let down our guard and maneuvered around him only with great caution.

Winter approached, and soon the holidays were upon us. I threw a subdued party for the nurses, handing out gifts and awards to the team for their spirit and courage. All the while, in the middle of the room, Harvey circled. As his brain shut down, so did his vision. He lost much of his ability to speak. One of the only words he could still say was his name. Our twenty-third wedding anniversary and my birthday went by as forgotten, irrelevant dates.

There was a deep emptiness in my life; sometimes I felt as if I didn't exist. Then in late January 2002, I received a call that there was an opening at Copper Ridge. Was I interested?

Despite everything I had endured, I was still ambivalent. What if it didn't work? My previous experiences with Harvey in the locked ward at the hospital and at the nursing facility couldn't simply be erased. I was hypervigilant, programmed to run interference for Harvey every step of the way. Turning off that intensity was impossible; I didn't know how to behave differently. There was also no guarantee that the doctors at Copper Ridge would be any more successful at finding a drug to manage Harvey's aggressiveness without dramatically diminishing what was left of his mental capacity. What was best for Harvey?

There were also more practical considerations. Would Harvey's nurses drive the hour each way to Copper Ridge? Was it a safe commute on back roads in bad weather? What if we were asked to leave Copper Ridge? Harvey's behavior was getting progressively worse. His doctor and my son Jason weighed in again and left me no options.

So five months later on February 4, 2002, we left the home we had shared for most of our marriage and set out for Copper Ridge. I closed the door behind me and refused to look back.

SIX

CHANGING LANDSCAPE

*T*he off-highway route to Copper Ridge passed scenic rolling hills and a countryside of red farms with bales of neatly cut hay stacked alongside. Winter parched the panorama, but the chill I felt came from within. Harvey had started drifting away from me emotionally long ago. Now the view out the window evoked the vastness of our imminent physical separation. Driving through this unfamiliar terrain, I felt unmoored. I felt like a failure, unable to rescue the man I loved. The road to Copper Ridge was a reminder of how dramatically the landscape of my own life had shifted. Everything looked different.

My friends had argued relentlessly that I needed to seize this opportunity. At times, it felt like a Greek chorus, dressed in black and predicting doom; their discordant notes echoing in my head. To be fair, they often put into words what I sometimes thought to myself but never dared say out loud.

"You've done all you can. You managed the nightmare and gave up your career."

"Put him somewhere safe and reclaim your life."

"No one deserves to be on call 24/7. It's not too late to move forward."

"Get out while you can before it is too late."

I understood the arguments presented to bolster their case that Copper Ridge represented a safe haven, not only for Harvey, but for me. The stress and the intensity of care that Harvey required—trying to anticipate his every need and keep both him and his caregivers safe as his agitation and propensity to lash out grew—took an enormous toll on my physical and mental health. I could never relax.

I often found myself sinking into a deep depression fueled by my growing sense of isolation. Even with nursing help, Harvey's care consumed all my energies. When I did leave the house, it was time used to run errands or see my grandchildren. There was no allowance in our budget for respite care.

The only time I was physically absent was for a monthly, eight-hour, same-day round-trip drive to check on my widowed mother. She was still feisty at eighty-four, but the problems with Harvey meant that I wasn't spending as much time with her. She needed my attention.

Recently, she had been in a minor fender bender, but when the police charged her for making a turn from the wrong lane she abruptly gave up driving. She no longer had any interest in walking the three blocks to the beach, even though watching the ocean had been her major source of comfort through the loss of both my brother and my father.

Even after she retired at age seventy-one, my mother had the exacting demeanor of a proud and independent woman. Always fastidious in her dress, she still looked as if she was headed off to teach class even when she was just doing chores around the house. Now she seldom dressed up unless she had a doctor's appointment. She let her blond highlighted hair go completely white. Unread newspapers stacked up in piles. There were other signs she needed help. She loved to cook so I had bought her a freezer, but she started forgetting her recipes and letting food spoil.

Over the years, her women friends had died off one by one. She had no energy to make new friends and refused hired help, even weekly grocery deliveries billed to my account. My mother made it clear she wanted only me.

So twice a month, I left Harvey in the care of the aides and made the trip to my mother's house to stock her refrigerator, clean the apartment, and take her out for an early Chinese dinner. Then it was right back on the road to reach home in time for my night shift. The entire time I was with her, I worried constantly about what might happen in my absence. She refused to wear a medical alert device to trigger the medics and declined my offer to recruit a college aide part-time. Visits to my mother came to resemble my trips with Harvey to the nursing facilities and the hospital; I never calmed down until I walked out the door.

I didn't always share what was going on. It was difficult to communicate the intensity of my predicament to friends out of fear of boring or losing them too. Each of them was dealing with their own personal brand of pain, so I listened instead and said nothing. Nevertheless, one of their honest queries gnawed at me in my darkest moments of self-doubt.

"Under similar circumstances, would Harvey do the same? Give up everything to take care of you?"

I never answered them, but I did turn that question over and over in my mind, especially as I drove to Copper Ridge. Harvey had never given up on his patients. I couldn't shake the feeling that somehow, in bringing him to Copper Ridge, I was letting him down. The truth was somewhere in between. For the first time, I was being forced to start considering what might be best for both of us.

Harvey had not been out with me in the car since we had brought him home four months earlier from the nursing home. He was agitated. I wanted to think it was just because he wanted to stay at home, but I knew better.

There was no turning back the clock now. Harvey sat in the front seat because he refused to get in the backseat. Both nurses hovered directly behind him, but eventually we all relaxed.

The movement of the car, the pastoral scenery, and Rimsky-Korsakov's *Scheherazade* playing softly on the radio lulled him to sleep.

Copper Ridge had a stellar reputation not only for its manage-ment of difficult cases, but also for the quality of their staff. A few weeks earlier, I had made the long drive alone to check it out myself. The staff-to-patient ratio was one to three, which allowed more engagement with residents. Unlike the aloof and revolving-door hires in other facilities, staff tenure there averaged five to twenty years. The way the staff handled patients was akin to old-fashioned country care. The corridors were twice the normal size, and the rooms were spacious. Residents freely moved around the halls many ambulating while seated in wheelchairs as protection from falling. The general population was elderly and docile. Aloud I wondered if Harvey would fit in and how long he might last. The admissions director then took me to visit the special unit. It was on a separate floor reserved for patients with the most ominous behavior issues of dementia care.

The ward was noisy and frenetic, like a raucous scene, down to bizarrely dressed characters right out of an old Fellini movie. The behavior gave clues to which part of the brain was diseased. Patients with frontal lobe dementia screamed profanities. So did Harvey. Other residents were calm one moment and then something . . . anything . . . might set them off in an episode of rage. That was Harvey, too. Still others wandered while hallucinating, picked at the air, talked to themselves in the mirror as if with a friend, or put foreign objects in their mouths, mistaking them for food. And then there was the repetitive, plaintive cry from those who could still speak: "I want to go home. Get me out of here."

Right before my eyes were the same aberrations I dealt with on a daily basis. Moreover, I got to see the trajectory of the problems I was likely to confront next as the disease progressed. I could no longer view Harvey's behaviors in a void. He was just a variation of them. The realization of what likely lay ahead stunned me, and I burst into tears of premonition.

The admissions officer suggested we leave, but I pulled myself together to ask if there was a place where I could quietly sit and watch. We moved into a darkened side room with one-way glass. The aides worked calmly amid the chaos. The hard reality was that Copper Ridge offered the best skilled care for someone like Harvey, but I still worried. There was so much noise; shouting and screaming often set Harvey off. The option to accommodate us in the quiet dementia care ward required the added expense of private-duty day nurses that met state of Maryland certification requirements. Fortunately, both of Harvey's regular nurses, Olga and Hla, were eligible. Copper Ridge also welcomed the presence of spouses, and I vowed to pitch in just as I always had. We would each work twelve-

hour shifts on alternate days to ease the burden and long commute.

It was early afternoon when we arrived. It might have been
a new setting, but we acted out our familiar ritual of normalcy.
We had dressed Harvey up in a sport jacket and crisp striped
shirt to make an entrance befitting a new VIP guest in residence. He wore freshly polished loafers, the footwear of choice
when you care for a man who might hit you in the head with
his fist if you take too long to tie his shoes. I refused to put him
in a sweat suit. I knew the dry-cleaning bill from his inconti-
nence would be high, but it was important not just to me, but
also to Hla and Olga that Harvey look like his trademark, polished self. They were the first to remind me when we were out
of freshly laundered shirts or when Harvey needed more after-
shave and cologne. They took pride knowing that they were
caring for someone like Harvey, a preeminent scientist, a doctor who had spent a career trying to cure people of terrible
diseases. It helped my nursing aides see the value in their work,
which so often could be tedious, frightening, and filled with
drudgery. They insisted on calling him "Dr. Harvey," and
they never dropped the honorific even as Harvey's disease progressed and he could no longer say his own name.

Driving to Copper Ridge, I overheard their conversation in
the backseat. They were skeptical from the beginning that this
new arrangement would work. As far as they were concerned,
we were headed to a private medical retreat to have Dr. Harvey's

medications adjusted, and that soon we would be coming home again. Still, hoping for the best, I arranged to be billed for snacks from the visitors' café to break up the monotony of institutional food, not just for Harvey but also for his nurses.

Harvey's room was on the inner court, two doors down from the nursing station. It missed the morning sun but was the only vacant room available. I had never unpacked when we came home from the last facility, so this move was complete, right down to the poster-size photo of us with Jason and his wife, Dana, at Harvey's induction into the American College of Physicians. There we were smiling next to Harvey in his cap and gown, but he was already having problems and his eyes looked sadly vacant. Just ten minutes earlier that day, he was confused enough to have walked the wrong way on the stage. Fortunately, the inductees didn't have to speak or I wouldn't have risked it. This was his last hurrah and I was willing to test the odds that we could make it through the ceremony. I mounted the picture facing the bed so if he woke during the night it might give him comfort.

I was always trying to imagine the world from Harvey's perspective and leave him clues of the man he used to be.

The room was not claustrophobic, but Harvey was becoming agitated so we opened the door. Off he went to explore the halls with the aides scurrying behind him. "Let's keep him moving so we tire him out," I started to say, but my words just echoed down the corridor as they disappeared from sight.

• • •

I took the opportunity to negotiate with the head nurse to let me stay the first night, recounting my traumatic experience at the hospital. All she said was, "Please look at yourself in the mirror. You're burned out. You really need to get some rest. If you don't take care of yourself, how can you ever take care of him?" She gave me her personal number and that of the night nurse, with an invitation to call at any hour, night or day. We waited through dinner and cleaned him up for the night. The bell rang that visiting hours were over. By now I was used to one-way good-night kisses, but he surprised me with a kiss back. So I did it again and again, hoping for the same response. There was nothing.

I drove the long way home, but despite my exhaustion, I couldn't sleep. That night, I called the nursing station at midnight, then again at 3:00 A.M. Both times, they told me Harvey was up, quietly and aimlessly wandering the halls.

For the first time, I was now physically removed from Harvey, but I got telephone calls with details of his condition multiple times every day from my nurses. Harvey was having trouble adjusting to his new quarters at Copper Ridge. Up most of the night, he slept much of the morning and was difficult to get up. Shower time required two nurses with him in a large tiled room with a drain in the center. They would literally hose him down at a safe distance with the door ajar in case they needed to call for backup. He couldn't sit still for activities or physical therapy. The doctors had weaned him off his current medications to start anew. It was trial and error once more.

I showed up on day three because it was my rotation and found Harvey sleeping in another woman's bed as she sat stupefied in the chair. I joked to the nurse, "She can have him if she wants him," as I led him back to his room. Nothing had really changed, except Harvey seemed to grow more unreachable day by day.

During the long rides back and forth to Copper Ridge, I had time to think and reflect, and I found myself doubting some of the decisions I had made.

In the seemingly endless search for a diagnosis, I used to take Harvey to the gym. I pushed him physically with rigorous routines on the indoor track and the weight machines. At each and every station, I demonstrated the routine, helped him get seated, and then assisted because he forgot what to do in mid-air on each repetition. I was determined to preserve muscle memory so he would not have to be confined to a wheelchair. But now, in hindsight, I realize that what I did was make him physically stronger even as his mind deteriorated. My best intentions had resulted in a situation where Harvey was feared for his strength and vice-like grip, fueled by adrenaline and aggravated by confusion.

We lucked out that 2002 was a mild winter, and soon the 90-minute round trip to Copper Ridge seemed routine. I went home each night to sleep in my bed and not in a chair or on an air mattress on the floor of Harvey's room.

Years later, long after Harvey had left Copper Ridge, the empathetic head nurse, Carol Palmer, told me that she did not think the constant calls from the private nurses had been a good idea. They kept me mired in the tiniest details of Harvey's daily life. I never got a break. Some things, she chided, aren't necessary to know. But I didn't get the chance to explain why this dynamic worked. I treated my nurses like extended family, expressing as much concern for their well-being as I did for Harvey. I knew better than anyone that caring for Harvey was a difficult job. They were encouraged to express their frustrations and feelings. I never asked them to do something for Harvey that they hadn't seen me do personally. These shared experiences held us together through the most disheartening moments that came all too often as tests of our endurance.

It was too late to go back and undo my decisions so I refused to dwell on them. For now, I needed to find a way to compartmentalize my pain. I did not get a chance to dwell too long on it anyway. I was always chasing Harvey.

Unlike amnesia, in which a person does not remember anything, Harvey suffered from agnosia, where he couldn't recognize familiar objects and faces. One moment he knew you, the next time he didn't. Aphasia added to his frustration and outbursts because he was unable to find words or understand

them. This meant that the nurses and I were forced to anticipate or guess what Harvey wanted or needed.

The Copper Ridge medical team conceded that there was
nothing typical about Harvey's case. None of the usual therapies seemed to work for his aggressive temperament and severe
dementia. Even when his foot got badly infected and so swollen
that he shouldn't have been able to get around, he walked through
the pain. I found myself nervously holding my breath each
time I walked into the ward, and only breathed normally when
I started the drive back home.

Throughout Harvey's illness, each doctor told me that, although the course of the disease was impossible to predict,
typically the downward decline of an early-onset patient is pre-
cipitous. They speculated that Harvey was not likely to survive
a long time, giving him roughly five to eight years to live. As
a consequence, most of the personal decisions I made turned
out to be based on a prognosis that was very wrong.

After his stint in the hospital, I had just assumed that Medicare would continue to cover his care. I was so wrong. Medicare covered acute episodes but paid nothing for long-term,
chronic care. I had budgeted for full-time private-duty nurses,
doctor visits, diapers, medication, and even special medical
equipment because the Medicare-issued portable commode
and wheelchair didn't fit a man Harvey's size. When I opened
the bill for the first month at Copper Ridge, the total for the
care and the private nurses came to $15,000. It didn't take too

much to do the math. My bill for his out-of-pocket care would run $180,000 annually. Here we were two adults in our prime and both out of work due to circumstances beyond our control. The fees to keep Harvey at a facility I trusted were simply beyond our financial means.

The situation reminded me of a similar financial predicament twenty years earlier, when my younger brother overdosed on prescription meds at college. I will never forget being rebuffed at admissions to Sheppard Pratt, a private psychiatric facility outside of Baltimore. They required a $10,000 down payment to admit him. It was money neither my mother nor I had. We had already wiped out our family savings caring for my father who lingered for twelve years mentally diminished from self-induced carbon monoxide poisoning.

When we walked out of the building, the ambulance with my brother came up the winding driveway. I instructed the driver to follow me and drove to the closest emergency room. Eight hours later, I signed my brother out of the hospital, laid him in the back of my gray Nissan van, and took him home with me. In the end, my repeated rescue efforts over the next four years failed. Long after his death, I often wondered if the outcome would have been different had we had the money. Now when I thought about Harvey's situation, the same questions haunted me.

Sitting on my desk untouched was the voluminous paperwork from the elder care lawyer. I was annoyed by the proposed strategy to shift assets and impoverish my husband so he would be eligible for Medicaid. I refused to take advantage of such a perverse legal loophole. There were families out there who desperately needed that social safety net.

I could divorce Harvey to protect my assets and continue to care for him, but that seemed like another obscene option that I would not seriously consider. Given Harvey's short-term prognosis from more than one doctor, I figured I could continue to tough it out for a few more years.

Nonetheless, it didn't seem to matter how I ran the numbers. I kept coming up broke in a relatively short span of time, even if I didn't consider my own future financial needs. Harvey hadn't had the foresight to protect himself nor us with long-term-care insurance.

Methodically, I started writing down all our assets and prioritizing what I would sell off first to pay for his care. The wine collection Harvey had built for us over the years was at the top of my list. What remained after paying taxes and auction fees might buy me not quite two years of care. But even this was conjecture, because I had not yet had the wine appraised, and the base prices were locked away in Harvey's head.

Each time I turned the key to open the wine cellar door, I choked back feelings of anger and remorse. In light of what was happening, I couldn't help but see the wine cellar as a testament to Harvey's self-indulgence and lack of planning. Every time I went down there, I seethed. Some days, I tried to hold onto the anger, thinking it might let me emotionally remove myself from a sense of responsibility for caring for a man who had been so self-centered. But in truth the fault was also mine. I had enabled and supported his behavior. Then I would recall how altruistic and giving he was to his patients. I saved one note from a long ago patient with unforgettable memories of the exceptional doctor he had been.

> *"Dear Dr. Gralnick,*
>
> *It has been so many years (1972-1979) since my con-nection with you and NIH. The beautiful baby girl I fi-nally succeeded in having is now a wonderful mother and teacher with three young sons. It was you who helped me stay ahead of the science long enough to render the patho-gen still and make this enclosed picture of two generations of our family possible. I hope somehow you feel the grati-tude I will always have in my heart. My thoughts and prayers are now with your family."*

This was the side of the man I chose to remember, hold onto, and honor with care. Everything else I locked away, just like the wine cellar.

At night, the fears did not stay in the cellar. I lay awake trying to figure out how to slow the financial bleed. The an-swer I kept coming back to was to bring Harvey home. What I discounted was my own physical and mental health. It was never part of the equation.

Around-the-clock home care was still expensive, but if I took a twelve-hour shift and worked part-time from home, I could stretch our resources for several more years. Over time the disease would slow Harvey down physically and even temper the violent outbursts as his mind shut down his body. I knew from my reading that eventually he would forget how to walk. There would come a time when I would no longer have to chase him or fear that he might elude me in the middle of the night.

If I personally managed the care, there would be no guilt that I was abandoning him. There would be no long drives in the dead of winter or worries that the nurses might quit. The daily fear that Harvey might do something to get himself kicked out of Copper Ridge would be gone. Most of all, I would be comforted knowing that Harvey was never neglected because of his behavior, never restrained or overmedicated.

I kept hoping that somewhere, deep in his dementia, Harvey would know my touch and remember he was loved.

All along my friends and family had been asking me the wrong question. When they demanded to know if Harvey would have done the same for me, I could never easily answer them. Who among us can know with certainty how we will act until we are in the middle of a crisis? I imagine that the doctor side of Harvey would have kicked in. He would have done whatever he could to get me the best medical attention and put me into the right clinical trials. But would he have abandoned his career to take care of me, bathe me, diaper me, dress me, feed me, cater to my behaviors and personal needs? I doubt it. No. I know it.

Over time, that point seemed increasingly irrelevant. The real question wasn't what Harvey might have done. It was what I felt compelled to do as a loyal and responsible human being. If I had once temporarily left him for indiscretions that insulted our marriage, leaving under the circumstance no longer seemed like an option. The timeline of the hurtful episode overlapped with the earliest symptoms of the disease and the vagaries of his diagnosis like a bad dream.

It was late December, just two weeks before Christmas. That day, I drove home from the office during my lunch break to pick up papers for a late afternoon meeting. It was something I rarely did, but it was not unusual for Harvey to be home around that time to let out our dog and grab a bite to eat. I hadn't called ahead, but there was his yellow Porsche in our driveway. I opened the door and called out as I headed upstairs to pick up project files in my home office adjacent to our bedroom. Suddenly the door opened and a woman I recognized from a work introduction, swept past me on the stairs and out the front door. Harvey stood in the doorway as I screamed out, pushing past him to check out the crime scene. The glowing embers in our bedroom fireplace were evidence that they had

been there at least an hour or so. Two glasses of now stale
champagne, the crumpled wrappings from presents exchanged,
and our bed in disarray were the final insults. His lame apolo-
gies only exacerbated the situation.

Only after three weeks of private anguish could I be in the
same room with my distraught husband, who treated me like
a time bomb ready to detonate. He knew me well enough to
fear my aloof silence. And I knew the threat of being exposed,
like a nagging conscience, never goes away. With one or two
calls, I could damage this woman's career and ruin her home-
life as she had done to mine.

For my own dignity, I moved out of the house on the
grounds of irreconcilable differences, even though we were
equal financial partners in a home renovation well underway.

My refuge was the small home I had purchased after my
first divorce. I had vowed to keep this Tudor retreat as an exit
strategy, renting it out. Who knew that I would need it again?

Jason had chosen to stay behind, unsuspecting of what
drove me away. So close to graduation, it made sense for him
to stay. I had given him the choice, but his decision was still
crushing. Determined not to let my decision affect our relationship, I commuted daily between houses to make dinner and
maintain some sense of civility, leaving after homework was
done. Jason didn't deserve to suffer because of our differences.
Harvey, already estranged from his own son, played along.

We filed for separation. Several months later, we jointly came to a decision, driven by the renovation, that required Harvey and Jason to find interim housing. We would all camp out together at my refuge. Our six-month truce stretched out more than a year.

Once again under one small roof with no place to hide, Harvey seemed decidedly different. I attributed it to the strained circumstances of our relationship. Like a reality show gone awry, it became harder to maintain any pretense of normalcy. There were episodic tantrums and periods when he would retreat to live among the dusty rubble and debris of our family home, now more symbolic of our marriage than the dreams we once shared.

But the timeline of this painful episode overlapped with two years of missed diagnoses and the fact that marriages are complicated. The cruelty of Alzheimer's offended me more than his infidelity. I just couldn't hold on to my outrage. I had been drawn back by his helplessness as the disease took its toll. I steeled myself not to focus on what had been lost, but rather on what was left of Harvey and how to save it. Unconsciously I learned to live amidst the pain and survive on captured moments of joy. I lived in the moment, like so many caregivers and family members who forget themselves in the care of others. We concede only to being stoic rather than heroic.

In truth, Alzheimer's had saved our marriage.

• • •

Against the unfamiliar background outside my car window, my lack of other options suddenly came into sharp relief. So a little less than three months after arriving at Copper Ridge, I made the drive there one last time. The nurses and I packed Harvey up. Then we brought him home again for good.

SEVEN

DRESSED IN BLACK

$\mathcal{B}$y the end of Harvey's first month back at home, I couldn't fathom why I had chosen this route. No re-entry for Harvey, even in a space called home, was without trauma and confusion. The new medications—a heavy dose of antiseizure drugs, comprised of sixteen Depakotes and four Ativans a day—did not reduce his combativeness. He was fiercely ambulatory and kept both hands perpetually clenched in fists so tight that his fingernails turned indigo blue. The nurses, so resolute that we could manage Harvey at home, now seemed less assured than before. We all felt boxed in by our conviction.

Not once did I consider how others might view my decision to bring Harvey home. It was irrelevant except for my son's concern for my safety. I knew how this disease brutalized families even more than the patients, who in time forget their plight. It weighed heavily on me because I didn't want my problems to inadvertently become his burden.

In the short time Harvey had been away, I had forgotten how much sleep I lost each night. Following his strange circadian rhythms turned night into day. I didn't stop to think what moving Harvey back home meant for my family. My three grandchildren, then ages seven, four, and two, were too young to understand why Grandpa Harvey walked in circles in the family room and never spoke to them. My explanation that he was sick didn't seem to make things easier. The fright in their little faces as they peeked into his room was heartbreaking. As an antidote, I helped celebrate every milestone in their lives and everything in between at their home. But I am left to wonder what memories of Nana's house they will share someday with their children.

Inevitably, friends and total strangers began to weigh in with opinions regarding my decision. Sometimes they celebrated my actions as a testament to love and loyalty to one's marital vows; other times they criticized my choices as self-destructive, a way to hide out and write off my future. I knew I was responsible and perhaps loyal to a fault. But my psyche was so scarred by what I had witnessed in the hospital and the nursing homes that no one could reach me.

Soon, my journal became my only refuge, my outlet for the mounting fear and guilt—a substitute for screaming out loud since no one who might hear me remembered:

I screamed at Harvey last night for the very first time. I was not gentle as I rudely woke him up so I could change the sheets for a second time that night. I screamed that I needed his help and I wanted him to scream back at me. But he just sat on the edge of the bed, silent, unknowing, unable to fathom my pain. I washed him up and changed his wet clothes while he tried to wrestle and push me away. It could have been worse. Then I felt so guilty because it's not his fault; it is the disease that is my enemy. I feel like I am disappearing with him into an abyss. I will never scream at him again. But where will the sound of my pain go?

Other times it was hard not to take our growing isolation personally.

We've been abandoned by others because Harvey isn't who he was, but should I be written off too? All I want are options to fight the good fight; options to seek therapies that buy us time and the chance for remission; options, even when weak, to let Harvey refuse therapy, to make peace and say good-bye to me. I want him to thank me for staying true to him. No one deserves to be forgotten in life because their disease is without hope.

• • •

If Harvey was going to stay at home, I needed more help. After ten years, I was emotionally and physically running on empty. I had already made the decision to hire a male nurse to assist us in rotation, but finding someone with medical experience, physical strength, and the right mind-set to be a team player would take time. And Harvey had to accept him too.

The takeaway from the Copper Ridge nurses and social workers was that if I didn't create the right team to back me, I would be useless to Harvey and have serious health issues of my own. I couldn't afford either of those scenarios.

The agency route for nursing aides was my last resort. The work required special training and yet they only received half the hourly agency fee. I was on the side of the nursing aides because, by all measures, I was one of them. Harvey's behavior disorder atop the dementia demanded continuity of care because transitions were fraught with dangerous flare-ups.

By default, Olga was our anointed team leader. Just five feet tall, she was spunky, efficient, and bossy enough to make her height a nonissue even when dealing with Harvey who towered over her. Olga had an opinion on everything. Hla, an infinitely sweet and patient young woman, had weathered the challenges at both facilities and bonded with Harvey in a quiet, very Zen-like way. They seemed to understand one another without speaking. Years later, after she left to marry and have children, she returned to visit him and tearfully hold his hand.

Word of mouth and friends with firsthand referrals also aided my search. I always had my eye out for real nursing talent and credentialed backup. But there were difficulties with my recruitment approach.

A friend of a friend referred a seasoned female nursing aide whose patient had just passed and who was looking for part-time work. I didn't want my home to be a revolving door of auditions so I arranged to meet her at a nearby Starbucks.

She was an educated, refined, and conservatively dressed woman in her early fifties who had been a live-in aide to her former client for five years. She drove, wanted part-time work, had taken care of dementia patients before, and demanded a top hourly rate of $25. In fairness to my other staff, she had to earn her asking price, and the negotiations began. She rebuffed the offered two days of paid hands-on training by my team as an insult to her credentials. I should have stopped there, but I needed the help. I decided to try her out when I was alone in the house.

We got off to a bad start. Testing my tolerance, she arrived late, missing our scheduled time to feed, bathe, and dress Harvey. She helped herself to coffee and settled down in the family room with the *Washington Post* while Harvey wandered in circles around the center kitchen aisle. I was taken aback but said nothing. Trying to lead by example, I asked her to join me to review the schedule for the day, but it did not seem to change what she did. Twice before noon, we had to change Harvey's clothes because she didn't toilet him regularly. Out of the house for an hour after lunch to market, I returned to find Harvey wandering around, again in soiled pants. Before I could say anything, she informed me that my husband was uncooperative. She added that he reminded her of a wild animal in the zoo the way he paced, rubbed up against inanimate objects, and never sat down. Shocked by her cruel characterization and lack of empathy for someone so sick, I made it clear her services would not be needed.

She threatened to file a complaint and sue for a full month's salary, since she had passed up another private client to work with Harvey. I called her bluff with a take-it-or-leave-it payment for the five hours worked and showed her the door.

I wrestled with whether to report her behavior to either the licensing department or the person who had recommended her. After all, everyone has their own standards of care, but I also didn't want other families with dementia patients to fall prey. In the end, I e-mailed my friend and delicately advised her to be more careful about future references. She e-mailed back an apology and admitted her mother died from untreated bedsores. In hindsight, she felt guilty that she hadn't been more vigilant.

That encounter was the first in a slow parade of potential nursing aides that I turned away. Some were not strong enough or too old to manage his behavior. Others did not speak English; thick accents are hard for dementia patients. Then there were the many aides who wouldn't or couldn't work weekend rotations or refused to pitch in with other chores related to Harvey's care. 'A number of the references didn't check out. When calling references, I asked enough questions to enable me to distinguish extended family from legitimate former employers. Then there were the prospective aides who only claimed nursing as a passion because no one else would hire them. They lacked empathy, didn't touch Harvey unless necessary, and seemed immune to the suffering of others. Not only did each candidate have to pass muster with me, but Olga and Hla had a say in our selection. Any new hire needed to respect and feel responsible to them for their support.

Just as I was about to give up on finding a male nurse, a friend passed along a reference and introduced me to Marvin, a thirty-five-year-old doctor from the Philippines in search of a sponsor and a job. He was well educated, reserved, and infinitely patient, and he engaged with Harvey during the interview. Having a doctor work with us also allowed me to slowly wean Harvey off the heavy regimen of medication, which seemed to aggravate rather than ameliorate his behavior. I helped arrange an H1B visa so Marvin could work for Copper Ridge in their research center while filling in for me on an as-needed basis.

Now I had backup and a skilled professional with a trained eye to monitor Harvey—an important addition, since there was no way to get him to a doctor during regular hours. Marvin had also studied acupuncture in China, but Harvey was too aggressive to attempt a session. Four months later, tapping into the underground Philippine network, I hired Dindo, an outgoing, muscle-bound male nurse with a positive "bring it on" attitude who worked on an intensive-care cardiology team and wanted a second private-duty job. My staff now consisted of four part-time aides in rotation to buffer me if one got sick or left for one reason or another. No one was allowed to do more than an eight-hour shift; I was the exception as wife, case manager, cook, and on-call 24/7 nurse.

We all took our cues from Harvey while working to support and respect each other. We did not focus on the inevitable disease outcome; instead we built hope and pride into each day.

I had read that the best male caregivers were ex-military who continued to live by the code, "Honor. Duty. Country." So I wove that sensibility into the way we cared for Harvey. Together we were a special unit. I lead the team by example and dignified our mission. We even developed a special code for certain unseemly personal cares duties—"Did Dr. Harvey give us a present today?"

There were weekly team meetings—debriefs to compare notes on what worked and what didn't. I was constantly testing new alternative therapies and dreaming up things to try with Harvey to extend whatever capacities he had left so the nurses didn't get bored or give up. Researchers call it palliative care; we nicknamed it Six Sigma after precision quality control.

It was comforting to have two men on the team, beyond just having backup for Harvey's episodic and explosive rage. Dindo was our master engineer at fixing things, while Marvin tried to methodically retrain Harvey's brain using repetition. But having men in the house sometimes made me uncomfortable. For one thing, I felt the need to be dressed and not in a bathrobe if they had the 7:00 A.M. shift. There was also an intimacy to the care that always reminded me I was Harvey's wife and not another hired nurse.

The first time I had Marvin help me get Harvey ready for bed still amuses me. I was using a Texas catheter that slips over the penis like a condom and drains out into a bag to save me from constantly changing wet sheets. Halfway through the procedure I began to blush, embarrassed to have another man watch me touch my husband in such an intimate way. Whatever vestige of privacy was gone at home unless I retreated to my upstairs bedroom office.

In just three months, Harvey walked nonstop circles right through a colorful hand-woven tapestry rug in the family room. We slowly weaned him off his meds, one at a time, and saw him regain enough cognitive capacity to answer five questions: his name, my name, where he worked, and the names of our immediate family and our long-deceased dog, Sash.

When friends suggested that I get a dog to keep us company, I laughed. I couldn't take care of one more thing. It only showed me that they had no clue about the details of my life.

So consumed was I about honoring and dignifying Harvey with the best possible care, I failed to notice I was beginning to shut down.

Our home went silent: no classical music—a ritual on early Sunday mornings with coffee, the *New York Times*, and whichever *Wall Street Journal*s had been missed that week. Off-limits was a night out for dinner and adult conversation. Once gregarious and outgoing, I felt myself become quiet and removed in conversation on rare times out. It was as if I had forgotten how to banter and relax. Color faded from my wardrobe as did the brightness from my eyes. I wore only black from head to toe like a widow. In many ways I was one.

Most of my closest women friends lived elsewhere, but they propped me up with steadfast support. Separated in age by a decade either way, we were all spirited and role models of survival. We had all connected in better times, but their lives had stayed on track, if you exclude kids in rehab, divorces, and death. Outwardly they were living exciting and privileged lives that kept them scattered around the globe.

They were my lifeline to the outside world, but alarmed by what was happening to me. As the well spouse and caregiver, I was disappearing too. They wanted me back with the living.

Each of them stepped in to wage their own personalized "Save Meryl" campaigns. Trish, my advocate alter-ego with whom I spoke almost daily, was adamant that I deserved a life too. She invited me to their dinner parties or events around town, even though she knew I had to leave early or might not even show. She joked that I gave off no signs of being eligible. I wasn't.

Time after time, Alzheimer's insulted and tested the loyalty of the few close friends I had left. From Paris, Michette helped me purchased Memantine, a booster drug to modulate dementia symptoms that sold over the counter for $200 per pill, but was not yet approved in the United States. But I regretfully missed her husband's funeral because of an emergency at home with Harvey.

Lisa, a documentary filmmaker and world traveler, rescued me whenever possible—luring me out for occasional quick trips to kayak, hike, cross-country ski, and share her passion for opera. She even shared her hotel room to help me defray my expenses and put up with my incessant check-ins to home. I missed her fiftieth birthday celebration and her Kennedy Center film premiere. Each time it was a last-minute emergency; each time we blamed Alzheimer's over a catch-up glass of wine.

The connecting link for two of my intimate friends was Lin, who had recruited us for her YoungArts board. The last of my fondest memories with Harvey are photos of trips shared with Lin and her husband, Ted, who attracted a fascinating mix of business leaders, artists, and celebrities.

All my friends turned down reciprocal invites to stay with me in my home. I got their message, and I loved them for it.

The most trying part of their rescue effort was my re-entry back to a lonely reality.

Not surprisingly, no suitor was knocking on my door. On the other hand, women lined up to offer comfort and companionship to men I knew whose wives were ill or had just passed away. The few men who kept in touch with me maintained a safe distance by phone or e-mail. One man, calling for a professional referral, became intrigued with my openly constructive critique of his business model—or perhaps it was the amusing start to the call, when I confessed that I might not be too coherent because I had taken my husband's meds by mistake. The intellectual banter woke me up; my circumstances shut him down.

A West Coast developer/golfer turned writer whom I sat next to on a shuttle flight from New York turned out to share mutual friends. He called me almost every week for three years. The attention was flattering, and harmlessly erased a bit of the void. Brazen overtures from married men, assuming that I was vulnerable, were both disappointing and insulting. I politely avoided their calls since I knew their wives.

Early in Harvey's disease, I did attempt just once to invite a gentleman over to the house for a glass of wine after I put Harvey to bed. He was a widower with two teen daughters. I worried about what might happen if Harvey started shouting or got out of bed. The baby monitor was next to my wine glass in the kitchen, and I could hear Harvey's every toss and turn in the room nearby. I kept apologizing. It was a disaster, and the visit lasted forty-five minutes. No sooner had he left than I pulled back the curtains to check on Harvey. There he was sleeping soundly on top instead of under the covers. Reflecting off the polished hardwood floors was a pool of urine: Harvey disapproved.

Most women I knew who did have another man usually had their spouse in a facility. I was never jealous or judgmental but very aware that they had orchestrated a life between the pain.

One time a woman friend called to share her excitement that she was seeing someone even though her two sons didn't approve. "Do you remember what it feels like to have someone who makes you feel desired and cared for?" she asked. Suddenly, it hit me: I did not remember. No one caressed my hair, touched my arm, or called to make sure that I was okay. I didn't hear the rest of her conversation.

Many a night I was wide awake and couldn't settle down, even though I knew I would be up again with Harvey several times during the night. I often reached for some distraction on the library shelf nearby. I began escaping into my own head at night. Nonfiction and biographies, mixed with self-help, fashion magazines, and medical mysteries, were piled high next to diapers, pads, prescriptions, and a panic button direct to 911. When longing for intimacy got the best of me, I attempted to write romance, a genre I never read, using a pseudonym and conjuring up men from my past.

> *Cabin of Our Feelings*
> *Madison pushed back from the computer and reread her thoughts. Not her typical style but accurate to the cascade of emotions when she let down her guard. They had been snowed in for a lazy day of love-making interspersed with the solitary business of staying connected but unconnected to their respective worlds.*
>   *. . . She had flown all the way to Bozeman, Montana, to escape her life and "live the moment." . . . How dumb to be playing games with someone she had known professionally for years but barely knew personally. And why had she sent him away when she wanted him close for company in front of the fireplace?*

My attempts at writing romance fared no better than they had in real life. At the close of each short story, I always insisted on weaving back to the reality of my present.

> *I turn into his warmth and once again am lost to his power, which is both commanding and gentle. . . . I feel lost, yet found. He is my Montana. . . . Then a soft buzzer went off. She reluctantly turned to refocus on the lost decade of her prime and the adjacent bed with her*

sick husband lying in it. It was time to turn his mindless and rigid body to prevent bedsores.

Even in the fictional world, I never allowed myself or my characters to stay very long in Montana. I gave up romance writing and shoved the half-finished stories in a drawer.

I already had one unreachable man. It was no comfort trying to fabricate or end up with another.

EIGHT

WE ARE NOT AVAILABLE
RIGHT NOW

One early evening in March 2006, almost four years since Harvey's return from Copper Ridge, I got a phone call from the retired handyman who kept an eye on my mother's house. Ziggy had known my mother for forty years, but lately, he said, she treated him like a stranger. When he went to check on her, he noticed her beloved *New York Times* newspapers stacking up at the front door. When he rang the bell to check on how she was doing, she refused to answer the door.

I had suspected for some time that something was going on with my mother's health. In our daily phone calls, she was growing more distant. When I asked about her health, she deflected the questions, preferring to talk in vague generalities. I didn't have the energy to push matters further. Ziggy's call flagged that my mother required my immediate attention. No sooner had I hung up the phone than my instincts for self-preservation dissolved into a crushing sense of guilt. It was time for me to assume the parental role in our relationship. I just hoped it wasn't too late.

I arrived early the next morning, after a sleepless night shift, to find my mother too weak to answer the door. I let myself into the duplex apartment three blocks from the seashore of New Jersey, unsure of what I might find and with the apprehension of every adult child who has respected an elderly parent's wishes too long.

After my father died, my mother had always insisted that she wanted to live alone. An English teacher with a master's degree in library science, she was well organized and her apartment immaculate. She prided herself on her quick-witted rebuttals to the politicians and pundits that appeared on CNN and C-SPAN, the two channels she kept on as constant companions throughout the day.

I looked around for telltale signs of disarray. Nothing was out of place. However, I was not prepared for what I saw next. The delicate complexion of my mother's elegant life-worn face was now tinged yellow with jaundice. The rancid odor in her bedroom confirmed that she had not bathed or changed her soiled clothes for at least a week. She kept repeating that she had no appetite to either eat or live. I bathed and dressed her, packed enough clothes for an extended stay, and trashed the spoiled contents of her refrigerator—a Pandora's box of poison accumulated by the lady who once loved to cook and now had forgotten to eat. I called my primary care physician, who agreed to meet us in the emergency room at Georgetown Hospital in D.C. The next call was to the nurse watching Harvey, asking him to stay longer.

I couldn't move my mother alone, so I went knocking on the neighbors' doors for help. It was an elderly community of seaside bungalows, and many of the residents looked in worse shape than my mother. A passing postman came to the rescue. Together we carried her to the car and nestled her into the backseat, which I had bolstered with quilts and pillows. It was a four-hour trip direct to the emergency room.

Ambulances and police cars blocked the entrance to the packed emergency room. The only way into the hospital was the main entrance, where I commandeered an orderly with a wheelchair to help extract my mother from the car. I knew the drill; at her age and despite her jaundiced condition, the emergency room would be a holding place once they hooked her up to an IV drip. The next procedure was the all-too-familiar mini-interrogation, administered by a senior resident, too brusque and short on manners for my mother.

"What is your name? What day is it?" My mother knew her name but was a bit confused on the date. So was I.

"Can you tell me the name of the president of the United States?"

Mustering the energy for more drama, she replied, "Do I have to say his name?"

The attending team was amused until I interrupted with, "Be careful. That's a political statement. You may want to leave it alone."

The nursing desk nearby erupted in laughter, and the senior resident quickly finished the paperwork to avoid further conversation. We would have to wait for a bed to become available, but it was clear she would need private nursing care. That duty was now mine. I got back home at 9:00 P.M., just in time for my nightly nursing shift. It had been a difficult day for Harvey without me. I ate dinner while the nurse debriefed me in the kitchen.

My mother's hospital stay dragged on for a week. The doctors wanted to wait for the jaundice to clear, but the nurses seemed eager for her to go. Her prickly personality antagonized the hospital staff. I tried to defuse the situation, sitting by her bedside whenever I wasn't on duty with Harvey. I recounted childhood memories of good times we had shared and pointed out that there were still years left to enjoy with her family. Despite the family stories, my mother seethed with anger and bitterness. I wondered if it was the creep of dementia that seemed to dismantle the social filters of her personality. Was she too tired to hide emotions she had always felt? I knew that she could not return right away, if ever, to her own home. I did not want to search for an assisted living center; I already knew the expense, and given my mother's difficult personality, I figured it wouldn't take long before she got kicked out.

Given the bleak options, it made the most sense to just move my mother in with me. She had never liked Harvey or doctors in general. How would she react living under the same roof? I wasn't sure if the fragile infrastructure I had patched together for Harvey could withstand this new challenge. Still, I knew I would not turn her away. She was my mother and deserved the same love and care that I lavished on Harvey.

No sooner had I made up my mind than Jason and Dana stepped in with a loving and generous offer to keep my mother with them until we sorted out what to do next. They knew they could not help me with Harvey, but "GG" was manageable. As soon as the hospital discharged her, she moved into their house. We even hoped it might be therapeutic for my mother to be close to her great-grandchildren. They called her "GG" and came scrambling into her guest bedroom over the garage to snuggle and play early each morning. Privately I worried that my mother's newness as a guest might wear off quickly. Dealing with MCI (mild cognitive impairment), along with chronic health problems, tests even the most close-knit of families.

We all settled into a new juggling routine. During a free moment in the day or around dinner, I would drop by to spend time with my mother and play with my youngest grandchild, Benjamin, who was not yet in school. It was then we began to notice that his little mind was on its own path in the way he played. The pediatrician dismissed our concerns, attributing the behaviors to those of a spoiled child and over-reacting parents. My advice to Dana, who had watched me battle insensitive doctors, was to trust her instincts as a mother. They sought a second opinion; unfortunately she was right. Remarkably Dana managed the intricate family dynamics with a cheerful spirit and talent that belied the pressures on all of us. A year passed this way.

By now, my mother was soon showing subtle but undeniable signs of dementia. Her growing paranoia that people were stealing from her or trying to harm her convinced me it was time for her to move again. My mother demanded to return home unattended, an impossible situation. Instead, we floated with her the idea of renting an apartment nearby so we could all be close. I couched the conversation as if there were options and the choice was hers. This was a ruse I had often used to negotiate with Harvey in the early days of his disease.

Together, we checked out independent living quarters at the best senior and continuing care retirement communities situated close by. But my mother was growing imperious and critiquing each place we visited. No facility met her exacting standards. She declared them shabby, even those whose faux-wood panels tried to replicate the look of a five-star hotel. In exasperation after yet another failed trip, I finally asked her directly what was wrong. She looked at me through faded blue eyes as she leaned forward over her walker and blurted out indignantly, "I don't want to live with old people. I want to be alone."

In the end, I moved her into a brand-new building in nearby Bethesda populated mainly with foreign college students and professionals who wanted to be both urban and suburban. I signed a short-term lease, uncertain how long the arrangement might last. Knowing that my daily routine might not permit extended visits, I paid extra for a one-bedroom apartment with high ceilings on an upper floor with a view that captured both the morning light and afternoon sunsets. I hoped to limit her wandering to a bit of exercise in the hallways. If she made it down the elevator, she wouldn't get past the front desk.

We decorated her apartment sparsely in less than three days. All the home furnishings had been buried in boxes after Harvey got sick and rediscovered like fossils from a life before Alzheimer's. We bought plants and a newly stocked toy chest for when Jason's children came over to visit. I also gave the front desk attendant emergency numbers, paid the housekeeper on the floor extra to drop by to make sure the stove was turned off, and installed phones in every room. I put my phone number on every door, written large enough to be read across the room. I made five sets of keys and left them in different places around the house in case my mother forgot where she put them. I also slipped a note under the door of each neighbor's unit with my contact information in case there was trouble.

Unpacking the cartons, I was occasionally distracted by the view out the window, a sunset that went from brilliant purple to orange and other colors that warmed the late afternoon sky. For a fleeting moment, I imagined moving in here myself and leaving my mother at my house with Harvey and the nurses. The sky darkened, and I went back to stocking the refrigerator.

Sorting out how to address my mother's health issues consumed me for months. Her doctors balked at running an expensive PET scan that might give her an official diagnosis of Alzheimer's, but her symptoms mimicked the disease and we assumed that was what she had.

Harvey's condition continued to deteriorate in episodic crises that left him even further diminished. He was now wheelchair bound after a bad fall that had immobilized him. A portable MRI showed no broken bones, so we did our best to rehabilitate him to stand for brief periods of time. He also lost the last vestiges of speech we had worked so hard to preserve. The doctors told me these were signs of the later stages of the disease. Harvey was still strong enough to throw an occasional and unprovoked punch, but most days we considered it an achievement if he turned his head toward the sound of our voices or was calmed by our touch.

Sometimes wanting to recapture the sound and vigor of his lost voice, I pressed the message on our answering machine.

Over and over, I heard him say, "Hello. Meryl and I are not available right now. . . . Hello. Meryl and I are not available right now. . . ."

I shuttled daily between home and my mother's apartment. I shopped for two households, bringing food, spending time, making dinner, cleaning up, and getting my mother settled for the night before heading home and going through the same routine with Harvey. Her paranoia in the hours between my daily visits and those by my daughter-in-law grew progressively worse. She imagined that uninvited strangers had broken into her apartment and stolen her money. She lashed out at me in rage, frustrated that she could not remember where she put things. Even when I retrieved a misplaced item, usually from the handbag that hung from her walker in plain sight, she insisted someone had stolen it. Her geriatrician recommended Seroquel for the paranoia, but we held off on giving her an antipsychotic because of the warned side effects. Instead, I lived with her delusions and incessant calls, knowing this was far better than trying to imagine where she was or if something might have happened. But this decision, made with the best of intentions, would soon backfire.

One day in early spring 2007, I was attending a meeting about the latest Alzheimer's disease research held at the National Science Foundation. My Blackberry started buzzing. The name Montgomery County Social Services flashed on the screen. Assuming

it was a solicitation, I initially ignored it. I eventually checked
my messages. A social worker was trying to reach me regarding a complaint that I was holding a senior against her will
somewhere in Bethesda. I returned the call immediately and
discovered that my mother had reported me. I brought her
doctor in on a conference call to immediately set the record
straight. Yes, the doctor confirmed, my mother lived independently in an apartment building with a family safety net of
care and daily visits. No, she was not in danger of wandering
away. Despite these assurances, the social worker warned me
if this happened again, the county would have to open a case
against me for adult neglect.

Less than an hour after that call, I went to my mother's
apartment. When I entered and recounted what had happened,
she had no recollection of calling social services. I believed her
but still reminded her that if she continued her behavior it
would be impossible to remain independent and live alone.
"Do you want your daughter to have a police record?" I asked
her in agitation but only got a blank stare in return. On my
way out, I pulled out all but one phone in the kitchen, but left
the signs up with my contact information. Four months later,
the police came looking for me.

It was the end of another long day. After dinner with my mother,
I put her to bed and waited until she was sound asleep to slip
away. Jason had insisted that we install a webcam in every

room. Initially, I resisted it as too personally intrusive, but it was the only way to monitor her safety. Installation was scheduled for the following week.

I drove home and focused on settling Harvey down for the night. He had begun to develop seizure-like body spasms that woke us both up. I had just crawled into bed beside him to massage and comfort him when the phone rang. It was 11:30 P.M. The local police department reported a 911 call from my mother. She said she was scared, and that her daughter had abandoned her. When the police arrived at my mother's apartment, she refused to let them in. The security guard gave them access, and they entered to find my mother hiding in a closet. My phone number was posted on the door, which is how I was located. I explained the situation and promised that either my son or I would be over to pick her up. Jason took my mother back to his home for the night, but I didn't want to burden them further.

I was done with trying to support my mother's illusion of independence. She was coming back to my house with emotional baggage that reopened relationship wounds, which I had buried as long-forgotten history.

The next morning, Jason pushed my mother's wheelchair through the back entrance of the house. "You told me I was going home," my mother said defiantly, but the home she longed for now was her childhood house in a Jewish immigrant enclave in Philadelphia. She did not remember the apartment on the Jersey shore. She asked where her parents were and when they would arrive to take her home.

I promised her that this was a temporary visit until I could drive her home, but first we had to interview someone to go with her. Suddenly, her gaze fixed on Harvey asleep in his wheelchair in the family room. No longer ambulatory, this is where he now spent most of his days. We tried to move the wheelchair to different parts of the house based on the best place to catch the sunlight to warm his face while he slept. He was not even aware of my mother's presence.

"Who is that man over there?" my mother demanded. "What was his name—the one you married? He didn't deserve you. I hope you got rid of him."

"Mother, this is Harvey, but he has been sick for many years. Just because you never liked doctors doesn't mean he wasn't a good man," I replied. "Remember how he helped us with Daddy when he was sick?"

I tried to change the conversation, but not before my mother asked again, "So when are my mother and father going to pick me up?"

Jason wheeled her into the dining room. Photos of the great-grandchildren were strategically placed in front of crystal wine decanters that I hadn't had time to put away. I wondered if she noticed the glass dining table for ten had been pushed off to the side to make room for a queen-size bed. I had draped the open archways so that she could not see the threatening stranger in the adjacent room. The nurses quickly learned to keep them apart.

After two days, I was already at my wit's end. This arrangement was doomed. No matter how patient nor how hard I tried to please her, nothing was right. I resolved to speed up the interview process for a companion caregiver who would live with my mother in her own home.

At first, I let my mother sit in on the interviews, hoping that if my mother liked the caregiver, the new arrangement might work better. I quickly realized this was not going to work. One applicant walked out after my mother accused her out of the blue of stealing her wallet.

I eventually settled on Maria, a woman in her midthirties who drove and appeared committed to making this work. She liked having the privacy of her own duplex above my mother's apartment. We agreed that either one of my nurses or I would relieve her for four days every three weeks. She seemed resilient and good natured enough to withstand my mother's rage. She worked by my side to bathe, dress, and serve as a companion to my mother over the next three weeks. Then the two of them went back to my mother's seaside apartment in New Jersey.

Maria tried to make the new arrangement work, but it was difficult. Before they left, I called the New Jersey police to tell them that there was an elderly female resident living at the

Margate address who had Alzheimer's disease, and confirmed that the caregiver in the house was legitimate.

Still, a few days after my mother left, at 2:30 P.M., the police called. My mother had tried to climb out the window and was screaming for help. On the other line was Maria. She apologized profusely, saying she had slipped out to the market while my mother slept and had locked the doors for safety. For an arthritic eighty-five-year-old woman, my mother's dexterity and physical strength confounded me.

I tried to reassure Maria that there was a settling-in period whenever an Alzheimer's patient was moved. I coached her on the stratagems I had used to try to manage similar behavior in Harvey. I suggested that she pull the plug on the phone before she left the house.

My mother refused to bathe or eat until she was so hungry she forgot to complain. Often, Maria was forced to retreat to the other room and wait until my mother's anger had calmed enough for her to venture back. My mother no longer lived in the present. She seemed most upset that her parents, dead for decades now, had still not arrived to pick her up. I felt guilty and upset for deluding myself that sending her back to her apartment might solve the problem.

Fearful that my mother might call the police or get into trouble when she was absent from the house, Maria started taking her whenever she went out. It was exhausting, even for someone young and strong. A ten-minute trip to the pharmacy often ended up taking two hours. On one such occasion, my mother started screaming for help in the middle of the store parking lot, shouting that she was being kidnapped.

A favorite outing to the Jersey boardwalk to watch the ocean turned dark when my mother screamed out to a passing patrol officer on a bike. Each time, the police were required to respond and report the incident even though it was easy to read the circumstances. I feared we were rapidly becoming a nuisance. After each new episode, we put new routines into place to try to address the issue. Instead of Maria going out to buy groceries or pick up prescriptions, she had them delivered. Outings were now limited to the small porch outside the kitchen area to take in the afternoon sun. Maria was getting claustrophobic, shut in the home all day with an elderly woman who often screamed. It felt like the phone rang incessantly. When I spoke with Maria, I could hear the frustration in her voice, and she sometimes dissolved into tears. I realized that Maria was likely in over her head, but I did not have the resources to immediately rectify the situation, so I focused mostly on trying to prop up her spirit.

A few weeks later, there was a knock at the front door. I opened it to find Maria in tears and my mother in the back-seat of the car. Maria helped me get my mother, who was shouting profanities, out of the car and around to the patio in the back of the house. My mother berated the young woman as I defended her. Then I raised my voice in a parenting tone:

"Mother, stop it. Don't you dare insult Maria whom I hired to help you. It is you who have closed down all your options."

Moving out of my mother's line of sight, I quickly debriefed Maria, though our constant and daily phone contact left me with no surprises. Apologetic but unwavering, she was at her breaking point and couldn't continue. She handed over the daily nursing book and all the receipts with the credit card I had arranged for her. Maria thanked me for not yelling at her. She didn't even want to wait for her final check and asked me to mail it. From her car, she rolled down her window to say, "I don't know how you do it. You're a saint." She backed out of my driveway and drove away to reclaim her life. I brought my mother inside and shut the door behind her. My mother was home for good.

NINE

BEHIND CLOSED DOORS

Once again, I had two Alzheimer's patients in my house. The dining room was still converted into a bedroom from the last time my mother was there.

The immediate issue was my mother's behavior. I could predict what would happen to my mother in a facility. Unlike Harvey, she fit the demographic, but she was midway into the disease and still fighting for control. Her meanness meant the nursing staff would limit their interaction. Personal hygiene would lapse; bruising or bedsores might be missed if I didn't take the time to undress her. Every time I resolved to test a facility, I got cold feet. Each time I bathed her, a wave of nausea swept over me for considering such a move.

I had long ago sold off the few remaining assets we had, including Harvey's wine collection. My mother's pension was not sufficient to cover the cost of a private institution. The only way I could stretch her limited resources as well as ours was to combine the twelve-hour nursing shift to handle both of them.

Olga, the only female nurse who might have been able to handle my mother's prickly personality, had been badly injured in an altercation at the nursing facility and forced to retire on disability. Dindo had already trained a hard-working young aide named Rocco to handle a shift. He was very conscientious and kind to my mother; she called him one of her best students.

So I made Harvey's all-male nursing team an offer. They would get a nice pay upgrade if they helped me manage the two of them under the same roof. I would still handle the twelve-hour night shift alone. They agreed to try out the new arrangement, and we settled into our new routine.

At the time, it seemed like the best, even only, option. After my experience with Harvey, I didn't trust the actuarial tables or the doctors' prognosis. I had been subsidizing my mother for years, never contradicting her sense of being self-sufficient. The metallic powder-blue Plymouth with a V-8 engine, which now sat in the driveway just to keep her happy, had been my gift. When she boasted to friends that she owned her home free and clear, it was I who had paid the mortgage when the balloon payment came due. I indulged her pride because she deserved it. But it also made her diatribes in dementia more painful. I was not counting on any inheritance as the only remaining child. I wanted to honor her by keeping her retirement free from scrimping to make ends meet.

Two Alzheimer's patients under one roof was claustrophobic. I felt like I was locked in a room with no escape. A good
daughter, I had always taken on chores and responsibilities beyond my years, starting at age ten when my mother went back
to school to get a master's degree. I was her financial and emotional anchor through every family crisis. Now all I wanted to
do was escape her. There was nothing left to give her, and
every time I tried, she rebuffed me. We prepared meals every
night using her own recipes, but she left them untouched. She
made unpleasant comments when she felt something wasn't
done to her exacting standards. She still remembered to say
thank you to everyone but me.

The focus of my frustration and anger was directed toward the
disease and not my mother. I couldn't help but wonder how
other caregivers were managing. Were they forced to choose
between the dreams for their kids and the needs of their parents? The advice that it was time to put a loved one away when
exhaustion exceeded the guilt ignored the circumstances of
their lives. What was the episode that triggered their breaking
point when they just said, "NO MORE"?

Long before my mother moved in, I had become increasingly
frustrated with the way Alzheimer's disease was portrayed to
the general public. I knew better than anyone that the thirty-
second television ads showing a benign image of a little old

lady with slowly fading, sepia-toned memories and a comforting daughter close by did not match the reality of living with Alzheimer's disease. Numerous nonprofits saw their mission as supporting Alzheimer's patients and families in the moment, but none could bring themselves to be honest about what lay ahead. In fairness, no one really knows.

My own experience made me adamant that there was nothing to lose in showing the general public graphic images of the disease, just as HIV and cancer advocates had once done. I wrestled with just how to do it. Unlike sufferers of HIV or breast cancer, Alzheimer's patients lived behind closed doors. At this point, I already knew Alzheimer's would win at home. Nothing I might do could change Harvey's fate. But I did start to believe that if people saw the real face of Alzheimer's, they might be alarmed and offended enough to band together politically.

Harvey had dramatically progressed into late-stage disease and an even more intense level of care. One night, I called the local poison control center with an emergency when Harvey ingested the mouthwash I used to clean his teeth. The simple act of brushing his teeth daily was now an arduous chore. He would bite the toothbrush or spit at me. Then one day, he forgot how to spit. There was no way to take him to a dentist unless fully sedated. Earlier, a visiting dentist at the nursing home advised me to extract all of Harvey's teeth. This was a not uncommon practice used with dementia patients to try to reduce tooth infections and avoid expensive procedures. I was repelled at the thought that Harvey wouldn't be able to chew his food and would need to eat baby food for nourishment, so I rebuffed the suggestion. Now I worried that he might be poisoned or get sick from the Listerine. Not only did the on-call nurse address my concerns, but she called back two hours later to check up on us. The callback was a comfort, but it also led me to realize how little support I felt from the Alzheimer's community. No Alzheimer's help center I turned to had ever called me to follow up, even after they switched to 24/7 call lines. I realized that when it came to Alzheimer's and taking care of patients, I needed to speak for myself.

Watching our financial portfolio dwindle made my anxiety level soar. I realized that I needed to get back to work. I seized the occasional invitation to moderate industry panels for a speaking fee. I shared the stage with many of the same high-profile guests I had once interviewed as a television journalist. When people asked what I was doing now, I simply replied that my husband had taken ill and I had left my career to care for him. No one pressed further except to say they hoped things got better for us both. I always smiled and thanked them for the concern. I didn't offer details about Alzheimer's because I was still not sure what I wanted to say.

Then I finally had my chance. The Alzheimer's Association, an umbrella advocacy group whose board I had joined, asked me to testify as a patient advocate before the congressional Alzheimer's Caucus, headed up by Democratic representative Ed Markey from Massachusetts and Republican Chris Smith from New Jersey. At first, I hesitated. I knew they would be polite, but I wasn't sure my testimony would make a difference. Members of Congress and the journalists who covered these hearings were used to every group imaginable arguing that their condition was the most challenging, the most overlooked. I wanted to somehow break through.

I worked hard on my testimony; every word had to count. Thinking back on it now, I admit that it was exhilarating to walk through the alabaster-columned halls where I hadn't been since Harvey got sick. The hearing room was filled with advocates; the expansive, semicircular seating reserved for members of Congress was empty except for two committee chairs. The hearing was being fed live on C-SPAN. Did close-up shots hide the insult of the congressional no-shows?

The Association staff had insisted on editing my remarks for the public record. They wanted the caregivers to stick to a narrative about pain rather than offer policy changes. In the end, I left the House chambers frustrated. This had been an expensive lesson for a newly minted advocate: extra nursing charges and I hadn't been able to say what I wanted. I vowed not to let that happen again.

Three years earlier I had met George and Trish Vradenburg, politically connected and committed philanthropists to the arts

and Alzheimer's. George's corporate acumen and inclusive leadership style was punctuated by Trish's charismatic charm and Comedy Central wit. We were all at dinner to broker a joint gala between two Alzheimer's non-profits. The organizations went their own way, but we bonded as best friends. Trish had a knack of making everyone genuinely feel that way, except when she was hounding elected officials to support our cause. Even then, they vied to be her dinner partner.

Time spent in their company became both my respite and refuge. Neither of them had ever known Harvey and sadly, there was no way to know him now.

They encouraged me to join with them—first, through a series of Alzheimer's galas they chaired for the National Alzheimer's Association, that over eight years raised over 10 million dollars for care and research. But galas lost their glitter and no longer matched our priorities. We were frustrated by so little progress on the research and political front. Together we launched an alternative, more activist series of advocacy networks, under the flagship USAgainstAlzheimers, and made possible by their largess. We believed in the power of US and our fight was personal: Trish to honor her mother and out of fear, George out of love for Trish, and for me, a desperation that Alzheimer's was not going to take me down too.

I started with a few personal articles, opinion pieces tucked away in journals like *Alzheimer's & Dementia*. I was testing my

voice, trying to find a way to convey the growing sense of urgency I felt that something needed to change.

> *No disease should be allowed to have as its victims both the patient and the caregiver. But that is exactly what is happening every minute of every day.*

I wanted people to understand the magnitude of the problem. The kind of care I gave Harvey was hard and labor-intensive and unending. I did not want my son doing for me what I had done for my husband and mother.

> *We have juggled work and caregiving, abandoned careers for part-time employment, been forced into early retirement, and jeopardized our own retirement futures. None of us think of ourselves as a martyr or selfless. We are just doing what needs to be done for a loved one. But what happens to them if something happens to us?*

It was a start. But even in those pieces, I never dwelled for long on the details. I struggled constantly between my feeling that people needed to see what happened behind closed doors and my natural preference for privacy.

Then, in the summer of 2006, I had an invitation to go public. Susan Dentzer, then a health correspondent for Jim Lehrer's

PBS NewsHour, called to inquire whether I would consider being interviewed for a segment on Alzheimer's disease. She had already reported on the science and economic burden. This segment needed a human face and a willingness by the subjects to let the camera crews into their home. I briefed Dentzer and her producer on the challenges for both patients and family caregivers. By this time, Harvey was no longer verbal. He spent all day confined to a wheelchair.

There had already been interviews in the media with newly diagnosed adults in their early fifties and sixties. I applauded their advocacy, but worried out loud that the public image being put forth by early-onset patients might neutralize rather than advance research funding. To their credit, they did not act or appear impaired so it was hard to understand the personal tragedy of Alzheimer's disease unless you knew the disease. In interviews, these patients were unable to concede how dependent they were on their spouses to get through each day. Their protective caregivers were reluctant to say anything more than a few tight-lipped comments that acknowledged that daily life had its challenges. After all, who among us takes away a loved one's last hurrah?

Even among Alzheimer's support groups, the unspoken rule was not to speak publicly to protect our loved ones' dignity. I couldn't help but worry about the reaction if I decided to let a camera into our home.

The only fresh angle I might offer was one rarely shown: the intensity and physicality of daily care. It made sense to expose the caregiving reality at a time when politicians were promoting keeping patients at home as a solution to Medicare's looming insolvency.

As a former television reporter, I knew the rules better than anyone. Once I let a camera inside my home, I lost control of the narrative. I would have no input editorially, no right to approve the video used in the final feature. I consulted my son and daughter-in-law, who were strongly opposed. They refused to be interviewed on camera or allow their kids to be photographed, and they threw out a series of questions that bothered me for weeks.

"Do you really want anyone to see Harvey in his condition?"

"Do you want strangers criticizing and second-guessing your decisions?"

"Would Harvey want people to see him the way he is now?"

As I wrestled with these questions, I couldn't help but think back to 1994, when former President and Nancy Reagan revealed to the nation that he had been diagnosed with Alzheimer's disease. It was a courageous act that gave the disease a public face and left analysts debating whether there had been early signs of disease during President Reagan's second term. I had watched that interview while seated next to Harvey. Out of the blue, as the doctor he used to be rather than the Alzheimer's patient he was becoming, he said, "This is a horrible disease and so unfair to the families." He was either totally unaware or deliberately in denial.

Nonetheless, after that one television appearance, Nancy Reagan had refused to discuss anything more. The public never saw the former president diminished; her devotion was to honor her husband and protect his legacy. The public could attach the name of the disease to a famous and familiar face, but the disease itself was still hidden from view.

There was risk involved in showing our life in all its vulnerability. Would viewers misread my motives for letting cameras into our home? Would families with relatives suffering from Alzheimer's disease resent the fact that I exposed demeaning details no one wanted seen? I debated the value of letting people see Harvey diminished instead of remembering him at the height of his career.

My reluctance to give up our privacy was weighed against seemingly overly ambitious goals: trigger a public wake-up call to the personal devastation of Alzheimer's and spotlight the crushing societal burden of the disease. In my passion to change things as an advocate, was I being too naive?

I debated these questions in my mind for over three weeks before finally calling back the producer and accepting to be filmed on two conditions. I insisted on discretion when it came to footage around the intimate care of bathing and dressing. I also asked that there be no video shots while I washed Harvey from the waist down or diapered him. Within those limits, the public deserved to see the harsh reality of the disease.

It was time to bring Alzheimer's disease out from behind the shadows of fear and stigma. Living behind closed doors did not honor his dignity. I had to believe Harvey would understand.

Even the celebrated PBS documentary, *The Forgetting*, which originally aired in 2004, never showed the real hands-on care. The general public and even families, who paid professionals to do the hard work, missed the details we were about to expose. Would my kids forgive me?

The night before the television crew arrived, sleep evaded me, just as it always had before I covered a major news event. The morning of the taping, I looked in the mirror and began putting on my makeup, but then stopped in the middle and washed my face. I did not want to hide the toll the disease takes on caregivers. The audience needed to see the emotional burden of the disease. I felt vulnerable without my makeup and the pain unmasked.

Fortunately in 2006 my mother was not yet living with me. There was room for only one story at a time. The crew arrived at 6:00 A.M. and spent all morning shooting daily care. Susan arrived later for the sit-down interview. The crew needed to move on to another assignment, but they were missing footage that captured the kind of trauma that forces families to put loved ones away. So the producer left behind a special camera on a tripod for me to capture those unexpected moments.

One came late at night. After changing Harvey's diaper, I was trying to get him back into bed when he slipped and landed on the floor. I couldn't lift him and he couldn't help me. I turned on the camera. I let people see Harvey, totally helpless in his underwear and splayed on the floor, groaning unintelligibly. The camera recorded me in Harvey's old checked terry cloth bathrobe, trying unsuccessfully to get him up.

"I'm going to try to get you up, Harvey," I told him. "Harvey, sit up for me." Harvey's only response was, "No, no, no, no, no."

At that moment, I didn't care whether I looked inept. I didn't think about how the room, once a library filled with wonderful books and now stripped bare like a hospital room, must look to a television viewer. There was no time for vanity or the normal considerations that once bounded my life. I wanted to capture the daily occurrences, the routine incidents and indignities that took such a toll on caregivers. Later, friends asked me what was going through my mind in that moment. I was not even sure. It had happened before. Another time in the middle of the night, it was a call to 911 to the firemen to help get Harvey off the floor. When I watched the tape, I heard the despair in my voice as I pleaded with Harvey, words that went unheeded because he did not understand what I was saying. "Harvey, please help me, love," I begged him. "Harvey, I can't do it. Honey, I can't do it."

• • •

I told only family and a few close friends about the scheduled airdate. I knew they would be honest with their feedback. Even those closest to me were incredulous when they saw our daily life on the screen. The reality was I hadn't even let them in about the full details of my life.

The professional television journalist in me couldn't bear to watch the two segments for months after they first aired, worried about what I would see. Nonetheless, telephone calls and e-mails arrived with a deluge of mixed emotions. Lisa, who had visited our home in the early days, called dismayed that things at home were so difficult. Trish and George wouldn't take no for an answer and insisted on dropping by.

The *NewsHour* segment triggered numerous unexpected conversations with people who recognized me from the program and thanked me for being willing to tell the truth. One day in the supermarket, an older woman hovered close until I noticed her.

"Alzheimer's destroyed my family too. Only after my sister and brother saw your story on TV did they call to apologize for not helping me more when our father had it. You made it possible for us to talk again. Thank you."

A nurse from Copper Ridge called, expressing concern that I was going to badly hurt myself. She offered to teach me how to use a Hoyer Lift to move totally disabled patients like Harvey.

A well-dressed man in his midfifties caught up to me walking on a downtown street to say, "Your story was hard to watch. Too bad your husband doesn't know how lucky he is. I don't think my wife would be as good to me. I'm afraid to ask and find out." Then he turned and crossed the street before I could respond.

On a shuttle to New York, a sleep expert from Scripps recognized me and offered that lack of sleep over time increases the risk of dementia. "Be careful not to become the other victim of this disease," he warned. I smiled, then closed my eyes. I had been up all night.

At a dinner meeting, a scientist to whom I had just been introduced, pulled me aside to ask, "Please forgive my blunt question. Are you doing what you do for your husband out of love, or are you just trying to do the right thing?" I must have appeared perplexed because he quickly added, "I struggle with this question myself, which is why I asked. My wife was diagnosed three years ago. The woman I live with is becoming less and less the woman I fell in love with and married. I fell in love with a person, not a body. How must my relationship evolve? I asked you because you have had almost three times longer to think about it. I also asked you because I believe you will tell me what is real, not what is 'correct.'" He deserved an answer, but then was not the time. I offered him my business card with a hug and a whisper to call me.

Professional women, most of whom I didn't know, contacted me out of the blue through e-mails. They both admired me and admonished me for sacrificing my career. A few shared the toll Alzheimer's had taken on their own marriages. One woman e-mailed me that she thought I was brave going public. She added that she would draw the line on caring for her husband when he either became incontinent or wandered away. Most said they did not plan to take care of their spouses at home.

I was mulling over the varied reactions when, one day, a woman I knew professionally called me and said she urgently needed to meet. Over breakfast at a neighborhood bakery, she confessed that she was struggling to get both her husband and herself through the early stages of his Alzheimer's diagnosis. No one yet knew that her handsome husband, a Washington insider, was in the early stages of disease. For now, at least, she preferred to keep it that way.

I listened while she talked, her croissant untouched on the plate. Then she stopped for a moment, her voice catching, and said, "I saw you on the *NewsHour* program." I waited to hear what she would say next. A few moments passed in silence. "I can't do it," she confessed. "I don't want to be like you."

Before she could say anything more, I stopped her. Amid all my uncertainty about how to move forward, my constant debate over the right words to use, I finally knew what I wanted to say. I told her, "I don't want anyone to have to be like me."

TEN

THE MESSAGE HAS
BEEN SENT ·

*I*t was a gray, cold winter day, January 16, 2007. The air smelled just the way it does before a snow as I drove to Reagan National to catch a morning shuttle to New York. The night before had not been easy. Just after midnight, Harvey had one of those frightening seizures that I had learned to recognize. It started with a sudden cold sweat and a glassy stare. Harvey's skin color turned almost ashen, and his eyes rolled back in his head. The hardest part came next: the loss of control and bowel function, as his body writhed and twitched. There was nothing I could do to stop it. The doctors had coached me never to try to restrain him. All I could do was turn his head to the side so he didn't choke on his own saliva or vomit, or swallow his tongue. Even though I knew how to manage the events, the four to ten minutes the seizures lasted always left me a bit shaken. That day, it was 1:30 A.M. before things settled down, and my alarm was set for 5:00 A.M. When I left for the airport, I was exhausted. I had no inkling that my journey that day would present me with not only an incredible opportunity but also the first stirrings of an emotion I hadn't felt in a long time. Hope.

I was scheduled to brief G. Thompson Hutton, Trustee of the Geoffrey Beene Foundation and CEO of Geoffrey Beene, LLC, on Alzheimer's disease advocacy. The introduction had come through Lisa, who had passed my name along to this southern gentleman whom she'd met at the Slate 60 Philanthropic Conference at the Clinton Library in Little Rock, Arkansas. Lisa's text was short and to the point. "If his office calls with a request to meet—JUST DO IT."

I did a search online but was hard put to find much information. I presumed the trustee preferred it that way. As it turned out, we were both scheduled to attend the Rita Hayworth Gala in New York later that week. At registration, I asked what table he was seated at and went over before dinner to quickly introduce myself. Three weeks later, a call came from his executive assistant with an invitation to meet at the Park Avenue Café in Manhattan at one o'clock.

I pieced together that Hutton had personally spent the past two years establishing and launching the Geoffrey Beene Can-

cer Research Center at Memorial Sloan-Kettering Cancer
Center. The Foundation focused on funding research designed
to lead to new therapies for all cancers. It honored the famed
designer, whose iconic career in fashion spanned forty years.
As CEO of Geoffrey Beene, LLC, Hutton had transformed the
global designer menswear company into a philanthropic entity
where one hundred percent of net profits funded critical causes.
It was an innovative business model—a unique positioning in
the highly cyclical retail fashion industry.

At this point in my life, I didn't carry a résumé. What professional good was an updated résumé with a gaping twelve-
year hole? What would I write in as my occupation—at-home
caregiver, case worker, accountant, cook, memory keeper?

My memories of the fashion designer, Geoffrey Beene, went
back to the early 1970s, when I did a short stint right out of
college writing for the style section of *The Philadelphia In-
quirer*. My boss also oversaw the fashion column, so I got to
open the garment bags filled with the latest fashions that were
sent her way. The outfits cost six times my monthly salary, but
I marveled most over those by Geoffrey Beene. His designs for
women represented an American version of Paris couture, and
a legion of well-heeled women collected them as others do art.
I loved the sequined football jerseys that he made into floor-
length evening gowns and his unconstructed men's suit jack-
ets, which conjured up the informality that came with power.

I thought it inspiring that he showed his collections on ballerinas performing theatrical dance routines rather than models parading down a runway. Beene had been a medical school student before turning to fashion, and in the office we used to joke that he must have memorized *Gray's Anatomy* to design his sculptured, slinky gowns.

By the time I went to meet Hutton, my closet was filled with dated business suits that I never wore anyhow. I tried to make do with what I had, carefully choosing a black cashmere sweater, slacks, and a tailored menswear-styled houndstooth jacket with velvet trim on the collar. But walking along Madison Avenue on the way to the Park Avenue meeting, I wished I had something more elegant in my wardrobe than just memories.

Then I got a reminder that no matter what I wore, I could never completely leave home. Two blocks from my destination, I received a frantic call. My on-duty nursing aide reported that Harvey was having another seizure and asked if he should call 911. That morning, I had instructed him on both the symptoms of seizures and walked him through how to manage the situation. Now I talked him through step-by-step what to do and waited until Harvey's seizure subsided. Still shaking, I arrived at the restaurant on time.

The chic, oak-paneled restaurant was surprisingly empty as I was led to my host's table on the far left of the room. With him was a petite, effusive woman with voluminous auburn hair whom I recognized as his wife from a brief gala introduction.

She volunteered they were celebrating a special day, but offered no details. It was not my place to ask.

Immediately, I was struck by their energy as a couple. After three years of marriage, they still behaved like newly-weds. Their hands only unlocked when it was time to read the menu. I found it charming rather than territorial and it set the tone for a more casual business meeting.

After the waiter took our order, we settled into a more focused conversation about the Foundation's structure, its mission, and a portfolio of charitable giving that included heart disease, protection of women and children, veterans' support, and animal welfare. Now Hutton was looking to create an initiative around Alzheimer's. He confided that he had received proposals from other major nonprofits but was unsatisfied. I talked about my personal frustration with the direction of Alzheimer's disease advocacy, which lacked the energy that drove federal funding for both cancer and HIV/AIDS. Hutton mentioned that he and his wife had seen my story on PBS. I guessed that was the reason for his invitation.

Just then my phone vibrated loudly enough for everyone at the table to hear. I excused myself, saying that I had to check in at home. I fled outside into the cold because the reception inside was so poor. My nurse was reporting back that Harvey was stable and he apologized for being shaken by the seizure's sudden onset. I thanked him for reaching out as a precaution and reassured him I would not be late for my night shift. When

I returned to the table, Hutton asked if everything was okay. I long ago learned that people didn't really want the details. I gave him my standard reply: "As good as it gets under the circumstances."

Hutton then turned his attention to his real agenda. He ask me whether I was interested in setting up an Alzheimer's foundation, to do on a smaller scale, what he had done with cancer.

I was unprepared for the proposition. I certainly needed a job, but I was struggling just to take care of Harvey. The idea of starting a foundation, setting up the infrastructure, and recruiting a board was overwhelming. He asked me to give it some thought and send him a proposal built around a five-year budget. The dollars on the table floored me, but so did his faith in me. Asked if he wanted a list of references, he said, "That's not necessary." I agreed to get back to him with a proposal.

I exited onto Park Avenue in a daze. I felt excited and frightened. Nothing good had happened to me in so long that it seemed unreal. I knew I couldn't possibly take on more, but I couldn't stop myself from thinking about the offer. I burst into tears, which immediately froze on my cheeks from the blast of cold. Outside it had just begun to snow. In the streets, the trees and lamps seemed to glisten with promise. Despite years of living in silence with Harvey, the dreamer in me was still alive. I now had a chance to be the steward of philanthropic dollars that, if properly focused, might be a catalyst to change the way the public viewed Alzheimer's disease and help drive scientific inquiry. At that moment, I wanted to share the news but wasn't sure whom to call. I immediately thought of Lisa and her hope that something good might come of the meeting. In a way, it already had. I texted a message as short and meaningful as her earlier one to me. "Surprise dream opportunity. Stay tuned."

Nothing was very different now from the circumstances that had forced me to leave my career twelve years before, but somehow along the way I had changed. I had the conviction and tenacity that came from personal pain. I set out to craft a proposal that reflected all I had learned with Harvey along the way.

My deepest frustration as an advocate was that Alzheimer's disease lacked the kind of activism that advances cures. There were some exceptions. Over the years, researchers came up with better clinical trial designs. They tried to organize more efficient ways to share data on promising drugs. Challenges to the FDA to allow more therapies to reach patients faster were beginning to surface from desperate families. There were growing public calls for making Alzheimer's research funding a higher priority through the NIH, and more support for legislation to help caregivers.

But at the time, it was a piecemeal fight in this country. By contrast, France, Britain, the European Union, Japan, Canada, and even developing countries like China and India, had announced national plans to fight Alzheimer's. Our country had no similar prevention strategy.

The demographics indicated that there were 86 million of us between the ages of fifty and eighty, the target ages for MCI, dementia, and Alzheimer's. Yet this generation continued to focus on how to turn back the clock and redefine aging. It was hard to engage people on issues that most of us preferred not to face. Hutton challenged me to think "out of the box." The new foundation wouldn't have enough dollars to fund research for development of a drug. Its 501(c)(3) status prohibited involvement in any political lobbying. But we could raise awareness about the need to identify people at risk for Alzheimer's, highlighting the importance of intervening before symptoms appear, with the goal of preventing what happened to Harvey from affecting others.

In the late hours of my night shift, between Harvey's night howling and diaper changes, I put my ideas down on paper in what slowly became the Geoffrey Beene Foundation Alzheimer's Initiative. I let my experiences with Harvey drive my proposal; what I had done out of love over the years supported my professional insights. Harvey and I were a two-person clinical study. There were lessons here that gave me confidence as I wrote. Our life together helped legitimize and strengthen my voice as an advocate.

Despite this, nagging self-doubt still haunted me. How could I take on one more responsibility in addition to Harvey and my mother? My care team worked because I was always available to assist. Taking on the creation of a foundation might upset the balance that I had spent years achieving. Out of necessity, my personal agenda was to sock away what I earned to make up for more than a decade out of work, and to replenish the savings I had raided from my own account to subsidize Harvey's care. But I knew I could not leave home or work traditional hours.

The solution was to set up a virtual office relying on a freelance assistant or consultants if a project needed it. I gave myself five years to make things happen. Then the money would be gone, and I would be out of a job.

I wrote a wish list for a dream team board on a Post-it and stuck it to my computer. Top picks on my eclectic list for their entrepreneurial, scientific and philanthropic boldness were George Vradenburg and William Haseltine, noted Harvard professor and AIDS scientist. I wanted Hutton to be assured that the new foundation was in seasoned hands. Sometimes I wondered how, from just one meeting, Hutton could be so sure about me. Maybe he was banking on the set of priorities that permits someone to care for another person with such a debilitating disease for such a long time. I never pressed him for a reason. But was this lifeline real, and would my proposal be accepted?

Harvey was my silent confidant as I wrote and rewrote. Sometimes I read passages out loud to him. I kept my computer perched on his feeding table so I could monitor his breathing, noticing restlessness or signs of pain. The nursing equipment that now filled the room cast ominous shadows on the walls and across the bed where Harvey lay sleeping.

Every so often, I took a break from my writing and sat staring sadly at Harvey in the bed we shared. By the time Harvey was diagnosed, it was too late for medications to manage his symptoms. I felt the public conversation needed to be about earlier diagnosis. Research should focus on finding drugs to treat people before signs of neurodegeneration appeared, in order to slow and stave off the worst aspects of the disease for as long as possible. To put it simply—our brainspan should match our lifespan.

A focus on earlier diagnosis could help drive recruitment for prevention trials. I wanted the proposal to reflect what I felt when I watched in horror Harvey's descent into dementia: the recognition that we are all stakeholders when it comes to Alzheimer's disease, and we are all at risk.

If Harvey hadn't been in denial, we could have planned better financially on how to care for him. He could have written down his express wishes on how much care he wanted and when to stop.

At two o'clock in the morning with the deadline in sight, I knew I had to finally let go. Hutton's invitation to move back into the world of the possible rather than disappearing with my husband into illness had sealed my personal commitment— whether he accepted the proposal or not.

I pressed the send button from my Gmail account. It flashed back "Message has been sent." I had no idea whether my ideas would be accepted. There was nothing left to do but wait. But I had learned long ago how to exist in limbo, caught between hopelessness and hope.

ELEVEN

OUTLASTING THE BRAIN

*M*y handsome, glossy black business cards, with the "Geoffrey Beene Gives Back®" logo in the center, bore the title "President and CEO." On the back were business addresses in Washington and New York. But the reality of my new job was very different. I operated solo out of a home office off my upstairs bedroom. There was no secretary. When tasks needed to get done, I did them. The arrangement allowed me to always be on call for emergencies downstairs with Harvey or my mother.

Even so, it was a relief to refocus my energies. For the Foundation, I had deliberately shied away from a mission of care support or self-help. For one thing, there were well-funded nonprofits who had taken the lead on those issues.

I believed that, given the sheer number of my generation likely to be diagnosed in the future with Alzheimer's disease, the Foundation could make the biggest difference by focusing on early diagnosis and prevention. Even as I respected the importance of care research, I was intent on trying to help save the next generation.

My hard-won expertise had come from years of trial and error fueled by a determination to battle each stage of Harvey's disease as the fight of our lives. Caregivers deserved to be validated and empowered, not forgotten. In truth, I could be an advocate on both fronts.

I knew how caregivers become the second victim; we just wear out. Early in the course of Harvey's disease, I had a painful bout of shingles. The doctor said that stress, lack of sleep, and the intense physical nature of my care for Harvey made it harder for my immune system to cope with illness. The bout of shingles was a warning sign; when it came to health issues, Harvey wasn't the only one at risk. Twelve years into Harvey's disease, I suddenly realized that it had been a decade since I had gone in for a physical checkup of any kind, including a pap smear, mammogram, or colonoscopy. Medical appointments, like everything else, had gone by the wayside.

My friends Trish and George made periodic visits to the Mayo Clinic for comprehensive physical exams. This time I joined them.

At Mayo, after informing the physician who screened all incoming patients that I was taking care of two dementia patients at home, I was sent to see a psychiatrist without requesting the meeting. I will never forget our discussion.

"Aren't you afraid you'll wear out?" the doctor asked me.

I told him I didn't let myself think about that possibility. Then I turned the question back on him.

"Will I wear out?" I asked. He had no answer.

He asked me if I had hobbies or a way to relax, and I told him that I did not. There was no time to pursue hobbies, cultivate special interests, or even relax by reading a good book.

The doctor likened my constant vigilance to a form of post–traumatic stress disorder. I was always on alert, and over time the toll from lack of sleep and hypervigilance would surely lead to health consequences. He urged me to find someone to cover the night shift. I told him I couldn't afford the expense.

Later, I took a cardio-stress test and X-rays of my shoulders, which constantly ached. My left shoulder was freezing up, making it harder and harder to lift Harvey. The doctor suggested shoulder surgery, but I did not have time. Today, the pain in my shoulders is even more intense, and I still keep saying that I will take care of the problem some other time.

My new position gave me the opportunity to walk out the front door. I threw myself into work, always looking to find a creative and fresh approach to promote both the cause and the philanthropy. My periodic overnight trips to New York for meetings with researchers, strategy sessions surrounding public awareness campaigns, and conferences on Alzheimer's disease were rewarding but also solitary. Several attempts to dine out alone at a sidewalk café right off Fifth Avenue and Fifty-Fourth Street, while watching the pickup scene, felt more uncomfortable than fun.

I never tried to make plans when in the city. I was just too tired to be social. Besides, I much preferred to spend my time on the fortieth floor in an expansive corner apartment, with a view of Central Park to the north, and directly down on the spires of Saint Patrick's Cathedral at Fifty-First and Fifth Avenue.

The place belonged to Trish and George who encouraged me to stay there on my infrequent visits. It was a gesture so personal and special that each time I unlocked the door, it felt like a gift. I nicknamed it Heaven. The quiet was welcomed; I felt safe. At night I left the blinds open on the floor-to-ceiling windows so I could awake to an impressionist sunrise over the skyscrapers. The light cast a warm glow on the parquet floors and across the library couch where I slept. There was a foldout bed in the library, but I never bothered to open it up. Instead, I just curled up at the very edge with a duvet and pillow, always on the verge of falling off. Later, I realized that I slept the same way in that exquisite New York apartment that I did when I was home taking care of Harvey. It was hard to live differently, even when I was away from home.

The way I survived professionally and personally was to consciously compartmentalize my work and what happened at home.

One of my early public service campaigns for the Geoffrey Beene Foundation, called "Rock Stars of Science™," treated top researchers like celebrities and paired them with icons in the music world. It was a salute designed to excite young people to consider careers in science. My pro bono pitch to the stars was that they didn't need to own the pain of a disease; they were standing next to the "Hope." Pulling that project together took me back in time, to when I produced live shows and worked against tight deadlines. The scientists' schedules were even more complicated than those of the rock stars.

Five weeks after Geoffrey Beene's "Rock Stars of Science™" ran in *GQ* magazine, the chairs of the congressional biomedical research caucus invited us to Capitol Hill because we embraced all major diseases. In less than eight weeks, I pulled together a three-hour congressional briefing and live concert.

Researchers turned up to testify about the lack of funding for basic research and the impact on the field of Alzheimer's. There were updates on cancer and HIV/AIDS, but the most magical moment of the day came when Rudy Tanzi (a top Alzheimer's gene hunter), Joe Perry of Aerosmith, and the director of the National Institutes of Health (Francis Collins) got up and jammed together.

At one point, Collins played the guitar and sang Bob Dylan's classic hit "The Times They Are A-Changin'." When Collins got to the line "Come senators, congressmen, please heed the call," with Joe Perry and Rudy Tanzi backing him up, the audience roared and the energy in the room was palpable. I stood on the side watching it all, not believing that my vision to honor researchers had brought this scene to life. For a moment, even after all I had been through and the reality of the harshness of the disease, I believed something could change.

But at the end of the day, after the researchers had gone back to their labs and the politicians back to their offices, I stood alone on stage at the U.S. Capitol Visitor Center.

There are always moments, as a caregiver and an advocate, when I wonder if what I do makes a difference. At home, Harvey couldn't tell me. In advocacy, one is never sure until years later that a project succeeded in opening a dialogue or changing people's thinking. As glorious as the day had been, the current stillness and emptiness in the room reminded me of life with Alzheimer's. Someone had to remove the signs and take responsibility for the final cleanup. Soon, I would head home too. The memories of the day were mine to keep, at least for now. But there would be no chance to celebrate or share what went on that day, unless I was content to talk to myself.

Things were getting worse at home. Three times in the past five years, Harvey's doctor had referred him for hospice care based on an assumption that he wasn't going to live longer than six months. I braced myself for the end and made funeral arrangements.

Unlike hospice care for patients with end-stage cancer, where the end-of-life trajectory is somewhat understood, Alzheimer's taunts patients and families in the end stage of disease. The more likely scenario is that the patient suffers a traumatic episode, perhaps a stroke or severe seizures. This dramatic diminishment is often followed by a plateau period; the Alzheimer's patient sinks deeper into the disease without getting progressively worse.

This kept happening to Harvey. Each time, the doctor ordered hospice care at home, predicting that Harvey would not live longer than six months. Each time, Harvey's health would painfully disintegrate and then stabilize. The nurse practitioner came to the house every two weeks to reevaluate him. She couldn't get someone like Harvey on a scale to measure weight loss, so she measured "active dying" by the circumference of his arms. Two times, we were dropped from the list.

At home, it increasingly felt like we lived in suspended animation. The truth was that Harvey had been sick so long that I had forgotten what he was like before Alzheimer's disease. Sometimes I took out old photo albums to remind myself of good times together, but Harvey's personality was no longer the same. He had none.

As the years went by, it got harder to recall who he had once been. I changed his diapers. I cleaned up his accidents. I dealt with his childlike behavior and unexplained outbursts. Somewhere along the way—even now I am not exactly sure when—my husband disappeared. I have slept by his side all these years to reassure him that he is safe at home. I kiss him at night and snuggle in close, like we used to do. If his eyes flicker open briefly—something that is quite rare now—I try to get directly in his line of sight. I know that it is unlikely he can still connect the image with the voice. I have no way of knowing what he takes in, but I do it anyway, just in case.

Each time the hospice nurse came to visit, I asked for a copy of her notes. I wanted to share Harvey's prognosis with his doctor, but I struggled to understand it myself. Harvey had confounded the experts at every turn. I never knew if this time would be different.

One of the most recent reports reminded me of the challenges of his case. Harvey was now seventy-seven years old and had lived with Alzheimer's disease for close to twenty years. The nurse practitioner wrote that she never expected him to live this long. For the past two years, he had been unable to hold up his head, had serious difficulty swallowing even when we massaged his throat, experienced seizures, and had a bluish coloring to his skin.

"He is so well cared for," the nurse concluded in her report, "that his body is outlasting his brain."

Harvey now spent most of his days in a specialized wheelchair, his chin to his chest, drooling, with his eyes closed. He never made eye contact, and he hadn't spoken for over seven years. He was losing weight because, despite our best efforts, we couldn't always get him to swallow his food. No one could tell me how much longer the situation might continue. Every time I asked, the nurse repeated the same line: Harvey's prognosis was that he would live less than six months.

I kept an emergency kit tucked in the refrigerator in the event that Harvey's seizures could not be controlled or he showed obvious signs of pain. The contents included medicine to relieve anxiety, atropine drops to dry out secretions, acetaminophen suppositories for when he could no longer take medications by mouth—even when crushed in homemade applesauce— and senna for his bowels.

There was one other bottle with a pearly salmon-pink liquid that I hid elsewhere. It contained morphine, and we all knew that it required a hospice nurse's orders. The drug was to be used only to manage extreme pain when all else failed. One evening, close to midnight, Harvey was more restless than usual. His face was contorted, and he made strange, piercing sounds—trapped moans from deep within that tormented me as I stroked his forehead.

I tried everything I knew to settle him down, but nothing worked. I called the hospice to ask for help. The on-call night nurse instructed me on how to administer the morphine by mouth and use Ativan as a booster to speed up its effect. If he did not calm down in the next thirty minutes, she told me, I would need to repeat the dosing.

I felt an overwhelming fatigue sweep over me after I administered the first dose. I lay on the bed next to Harvey, trying to comfort him by tracing circles with my index finger right at the base of his neck. Nothing was working. The nurse called to check on us thirty minutes later. She told me I needed to give him another dose. His breathing was shallow. Resting my head on my chest, I obsessed over his every moan. Harvey's face had always been a road map for us, letting us know if he was suffering even when he could no longer speak. Now his face offered no information about what might come next. I kept listening for a heartbeat.

Lying there, my thoughts drifted to an encounter I had had a few years earlier after giving a speech at a conference in Boston. This was part of my new life and job representing the Geoffrey Beene Foundation Alzheimer's Initiative. I shared not only a vision for the future of Alzheimer's research but also parts of my story, so the audience could understand why I felt it was so important to develop tools to identify high-risk people before they manifested symptoms of Alzheimer's disease. It wasn't easy sharing something so deeply personal. Often, after I talked, people in the audience came up to me with their own tales.

A man in a motorized wheelchair approached me after this particular talk. "You know that your husband would not consider this living, and he wouldn't want you trapped either," he told me. He asked for my card and said he would call me to continue our conversation some other time.

Less than a week later, the call came. At first, I assumed he was just lonely and wanted someone to listen. He described how his life had changed when he was paralyzed from the waist down in a motorcycle accident when much younger. His interests centered on end-of-life considerations. He shared in detail, without my request and to my horror, how to use a plastic bag to assist someone to die. The helium gas tank that I often bought to fill balloons at birthday parties would be lethal when turned on inside a plastic bag secured firmly enough not to leak.

This was the side of being an advocate that always haunted me. As the main caregiver for Harvey, I made decisions for him every day without any advice, since he had left no specific instructions. Even when he could no longer say my name, I felt he trusted me and knew I was there. When he was in pain, no one knew better than I how to adjust his body and comfort him.

Yet in my role as advocate, I was questioned all the time. People I didn't know heard me talk and felt that they knew me. They debated my choices, second-guessed my decisions. They called me late at night to talk or offer unsolicited advice.

But here tonight, with Harvey's breathing getting shallower and shallower, and during many similar crises over the years, I realized that I was alone. Being an advocate hadn't changed this essential reality of my life. Lying on the bed next to Harvey, I was the one on guard. I couldn't help but wonder when Harvey's brain, having forgotten almost everything else, would simply forget how to breathe.

• • •

Harvey survived the night. The disease did not seem to want to let him go. The following day, I was scheduled to announce the winner of the Geoffrey Beene Global NeuroDiscovery Challenge at the Alzheimer's Global Summit in New York. I didn't want to cancel, but I was also shaken by the previous evening's events. There had been similar incidents in the past. Each time Harvey had surprised the doctors as he just sunk deeper and more diminished into the disease.

Over the last five months, I had been working on the details of an online innovation challenge, which posed a perplexing question: Why are women more at risk for Alzheimer's disease than men? I knew the statistics well. Women are twice as likely as men to get Alzheimer's disease, and we represent two-thirds of patients because we live longer. Those of us who do not get the disease are likely to be the primary caregivers for someone who has it. I was intrigued by a Mayo Clinic study on aging that had also shown differences between women and men in the onset, course, and presentation of Alzheimer's.

Sometimes, in those dark hours waiting to see if Harvey would continue to breathe, I thought about my own risks. I knew that because my mother has Alzheimer's disease, I was most likely at higher risk. The latest research even indicated that inheritance of Alzheimer's was stronger when it came from the mother's side than the father's. Women also reportedly progress faster from mild cognitive impairment into full-blown Alzheimer's than men—perhaps the reason Harvey was able to hide out for years.

What might Alzheimer's research look like if science and advocacy coalesced to crowdsource such a challenge to a global network of millions of problem solvers and experts worldwide? Why not apply innovative tools from global investigators in multiple disciplines of medical science, as well as engineering, computer science, and mathematics, to elucidate the effects of sex differences on the development of the disease? Both women and men would benefit. What better way to mobilize women than by asking a question that mattered to them?

This rigorous scientific challenge, with $100,000 in awards, had already exceeded expectations in terms of both scientific interest and global outreach, with more than eight hundred open project rooms from sixty-five countries. How could I miss this awards session? I had carefully orchestrated every element, down to betting on the wisdom of the crowd by inviting ordinary citizens to vote online alongside the scientific community for the winning submission. The results of the on-line finals had attracted 6,500 votes from thirty-six countries in just five days. Wouldn't Harvey want me to go? I owed it to the Foundation's donor to see this project wrapped up the right way. I whispered in Harvey's ear to wait for me and walked out the door, precisely as the morning nurse arrived for duty.

That afternoon, at the New York Academy of Science, I stood before five hundred world-renowned scientists at the Global

CEO initiative on Alzheimer's and conceded that there was nothing more I could do to help my husband or others already struggling with the disease. The focus must now be on a new conversation around prevention. I saluted the passion for science shared by all researchers by relating a story about Harvey's long descent into Alzheimer's; how he dragged two bulging briefcases filled with research papers everywhere he went. One day, trying to get him to stop walking in circles, I picked up one of his early published research papers and began to read it aloud. I didn't understand what I read, but the words caught Harvey's attention. I kept reading, but with each line I lowered my voice. To hear me, he had to come closer. It took thirty minutes, but he ended up sitting next to me as I read and reread the pages. It was a breakthrough; a way into his psyche. The depth of his passion for science was intact even though he had long forgotten my name. Even without words, Harvey had taught me the power of discovery—the way it inspires those who give themselves over to research and who never give up in their search to save lives.

Heading home that night after the event, I realized something in my own life had changed. Harvey had made it through one more day in relative comfort, but the events that transpired the night before were disturbingly different. For the first time, I started to focus on the possibility that the end might be near.

REPEATING MYSELF

*O*nce again, I sit in a tiny office, filling out papers and answering questions. Everything seems familiar. There are questions about whether I have noticed any changes in behavior. These are tests to see if there are issues with memory. The appointment is at Massachusetts General Hospital's Alzheimer's Research Center. But there is one major difference. The appointment is not for Harvey. It is for me.

I feel ambivalent about my presence in this room—not the caregiver today but the potential future patient. I have signed up to participate in an Alzheimer's longitudinal study. As a volunteer, I will be tested once a year. Psychologists will probe to see if my memory is waning. Doctors will analyze my blood and urine for markers of impending disease. I like to think by contributing my data that I am making a difference. If enough people participate in this and other similar studies, then scientists will be able to find patterns and make discoveries. Perhaps they will use the data to test drugs or find ways to intervene earlier; hopefully Alzheimer's will not cloud the next generation.

Nonetheless, even after all I have been through, I feel worried about someone testing my cognitive abilities. I want reassurance, but under the terms of the study protocol, I will not get any. Even if I show some early sign of the disease that affects Harvey and my mother, the clinical team cannot share the information with me.

Knowing this, I might have chosen another way to allay my personal fears, but outside of joining a study, testing is an expensive proposition. It requires a battery of tests, including a special type of PET scan. My personal physician could access these procedures for me, but the cost of the scan alone is around $3,000 out of pocket. The expense seems frivolous when there is nothing to do but live with anything the tests reveal. I would rather participate in a study so that my data helps move the science forward.

My anxieties help me understand why it is so difficult to recruit for large-scale Alzheimer's prevention studies and trials. I sit in this uncomfortable metal chair hoping that I will notice if, year-to-year, there is a change in how many words on the list I can remember, or how quickly I answer the doctors' questions.

One of the biggest obstacles for me personally was the requirement that I be accompanied today by an "informant," an unsettling term the researchers use for someone who knows you well enough to spot changes in your activities or behavior and agrees to come with you each time to give a report.

I understand the reasoning behind this request but balk at the idea. Any viewpoint this person has is highly subjective. Moreover, knowing that someone is always peering over my shoulder is likely to change the dynamic of a relationship. The condition leads to another realization. My women friends don't see me frequently enough to be able to fulfill this role. I certainly don't want my son or his wife to question my every move. So who is left? I am truly on this journey alone.

Earlier that morning, I grabbed the 6:30 shuttle to come to Boston for the testing. I even put in a 4:00 A.M. reminder to the nurse who usually comes at 7:30 to replace me.

I continue to push myself hard, even as Harvey wastes away. His legs are now the size of my arms and his rib cage skeletal. The nurses are amazed that his body has not returned to a fetal position as it shuts down, but we continue to stretch him several times a day and uncurl his fingers rather than letting them knot up into fists.

Given how ill Harvey is, there is a do-not-resuscitate order in place. I run through the other parts of the protocol with the nurses to follow in my absence. There will be no 911 call. The first call is to hospice. There will be no feeding tubes, and he will be kept at home whatever happens.

Others who have lost loved ones to Alzheimer's have admitted to me privately that, as hard as they try, all they remember is the agonizing end. Perhaps they had anticipated a sense of relief that it was finally over and were surprised to feel the grief of loss. I try not to think too much about it.

The study session begins with a short preliminary interview in a small, claustrophobic cubicle that only has room for two bodies and a desk. The first series of questions make me feel like I'm in the wrong clinic. I have listed "caregiver" as my occupation.

"Do you have any hobbies?" If I did, I don't have them now. No time.

"Do you find yourself depressed at times and drawing away from social interaction?" I feel endless sadness. I'm too worn out to be social, so I tell myself it doesn't matter.

"What do you do for pleasure?" I try to spend time with my grandchildren. I escape to their world from time to time. They say I wear black too much. I agree.

I think most people are worried about their own risk if they have seen Alzheimer's in their family. I worry all the time. When I walk up the steps to retrieve something and pause to try to remember what it was, I fear that I have begun to slip. When

I mistakenly walk out without my house keys or misplace my jewelry or money tucked away for safekeeping, I panic. Is this the beginning? Can my forgetfulness be explained by a genetic effect?

Other memories are so vivid that I feel as if they happened just yesterday. I remember every detail of when my son was born forty-four years ago and every detail of the day Harvey and I met. At the same time, I try hard to forget how difficult my journey has been. For one thing, it is not yet over. Besides, I refuse to complain because I just see pain everywhere.

There is the day I go to a doctor's appointment. The elevator door opens for a woman clutching medical charts followed by her husband moving stiffly and slowly. I empathize with her immediately. I can tell she is impatient. I identify with the sense of exasperation that rises up unbidden and is hard to quell, even when you love someone.

One evening out at the neighborhood Chinese restaurant, I overhear a couple in the booth behind me quietly arguing when the husband asks his wife where to sign the check. The wife accuses him of drinking too much. I lose my appetite because Harvey and I were once very much like that couple. She, too, may be missing the earliest of warning signs for Alzheimer's.

On the few occasions when I go out, I try to leave the disease behind and feign normalcy. This attempt rarely succeeds.

There are some days when I am convinced that my life will always be confined by Alzheimer's.

As I move through a reception or party of friends and strangers, I am alert for subtle telltale signs of the disease.

Lately, I find they are everywhere. On a rare night out to dinner, I find myself wondering what lies ahead for the man who asks me to check on his wife in the ladies' room because she has been away too long.

I can't take my eyes off a woman who stands lost and staring at the buffet table, uncertain and confused about how to navigate or where to start. I feel a wave of sadness and recognition when she returns to her seat with an empty plate.

In cocktail conversation, I am aware of a gentleman filling in words as his wife recounts their family vacation but can't recall where they went. They'd just returned two days earlier.

At a ninetieth birthday party at a country club for a community business leader about to embark on a solo trip to Madagascar, I marvel at his eloquence and his still-sharp mind. Over the course of the evening, I am introduced to three men in their midseventies, dapper and tan longtime golfing buddies. One man keeps repeating a story about a recent high-profile business deal, except the outcome keeps changing. No one seems to notice, or if they do, it's attributed to too much alcohol during a festive evening.

One encounter or episode may mean nothing. Perhaps the

confusion is simply the result of drug interactions, stress, or not enough sleep. Any suggestion that it might be wise to see a neurologist if this pattern of behavior continues will likely be taken the wrong way. Even when I am almost certain there is an issue, I am at a loss for how to begin such a personal conversation. Doctors aren't very good at it either, and it's their job to deliver hard news.

I think I would feel negligent about my silence if there were some early intervention or disease-modifying therapy that might buy more intelligible time, but there are still none. So I err on the side of being polite and say nothing, and wonder once I return home if I am doing them—doing all of us—a disservice by not speaking up.

I used to think of myself as the well spouse, but now I realize this isn't the case. My vulnerabilities are great. Any hint of forgetting, whether real or not, gnaws at me. I want to believe that I will know what to do and not be robbed of that final act of control. But when I look around me, I can't help but think this won't be the case.

My mother used to squirrel away prescription drugs. When I confronted her about what she was doing, she always replied, "What happened to your husband won't happen to me. I'll take care of it. That's not living!" But Alzheimer's often robs people of their abilities in an incremental fashion; few of us know when too much has been lost. My mother never used those drugs, and now her mind is too demented to have a say about deciding when enough is enough.

Each time I bathe and feed my mother, I fear for myself. I used to pride myself on being well organized and meticulous like my mother, but now I look at my cluttered desk and feel like I live in a state of chronic disarray. It was one of the first symptoms that something was wrong with Harvey. That makes me worry even more. Sometimes I can't retrieve a document, even when I file it away for safekeeping.

Experts say the barrage of incoming e-mails, phone calls, and texts taxes the prefrontal cortex, inhibiting the brain's ability to focus. Some of us can handle the overload, but most cannot. That thought doesn't make me feel any better.

If I begin to sleep, I never fully rest. Perhaps that's why I have trouble concentrating and review my work over and over. Researchers tell me that as once-robust networks of nerve cells start to weaken and connections get lost, it gets harder to remember things and keep track of people, objects, and events. At this point, I assume that my hippocampus—a hub of 100 billion nerve cells deep in the brain that helps make and store memories—is too worn out to activate and encode new memories or ever grow new nerve cells again?

My ability to remember things like names and faces stumps me more often than not. I've read it is a problem of retrieval and not storage—misplaced but not missing. I like to think I can compensate with lists and mnemonic triggers, but I still misplace my keys and now seem to be forgetting how to spell. That's not a good sign for a former school spelling champion.

These days I blame it all on the stress that seems to blanket my brain. Stress was the first explanation given for my husband's erratic behavior and moods. Now it, along with a heightened sense of vigilance, are the emotions I most keenly feel. My efforts to resist comfort food when I am tired at night are not working. My prescription for antidepressants needs to be refilled. I keep forgetting to reorder. Or am I just too busy?

At Mass General, the psychologist hands me pen and paper, and I prepare for the next test. I am a little surprised that I can't seem to control my anxiety. No one except the researchers will see my test results.

I already went public several years ago, opening my genetic profile test results on camera on ABC's *Nightline*. Anchor Terry Moran and I went through the genetic testing experience together to open up a dialogue about the potential risks and benefits of knowing your predisposition to a disease when there are no cures.

As one of nine children of a mother with early-onset Alzheimer's, Terry was relieved by his results. I, on the other hand, found out that I have one of the genetic markers that researchers say is associated with increased risk of getting Alzheimer's disease. I did not worry about sharing the information on television. I had already let television cameras inside my home to see life with Harvey; it seemed less invasive to let them film me opening an envelope that contained results I had long assumed anyway. But I will never forget my son's reaction. No sooner had the piece aired than the phone rang. It was my son shouting. "Mom, what the hell did you just do?" he asked me. "You'll never be able to get health insurance."

I had told Jason that I was doing a television feature and that I was taking the test. He later admitted that he hadn't considered the impact until he saw the program. I understood his reaction. Fear of repercussions is why many people refuse to get tested. In almost every circumstance, I consider myself a very private person. The only reason I agreed to go public was to try to spark an important conversation.

I believe knowing my risk lets me prioritize what's important. I want to get my life in order now while I can still make decisions and plans that neither Harvey nor my mother got to make.

I have two long-term-care policies. Unlike Harvey, I've left clear directives about what to do if I am incapacitated by Alzheimer's disease. I want to be cared for at home, in my own home, not a facility. If I can no longer lift my hand to feed myself, I don't want to be fed or given water. This hopefully guarantees that I will not live with Alzheimer's for very long. I do not think Jason will feel comfortable with my decision, but being a burden haunts me more than death.

The images of Jason I hold close are the best of my memories. Dana is tolerant when I call exactly at 8:10 A.M. on his birthday to wake him on the moment he was born. I marvel at the authentic man he has become, but I am not sure what he will remember or cherish most about me.

We were alone together for most of his early years. Now when I watch him enjoy his children at play or indulge them with tennis and riding lessons that I could never afford, I regret that I left him an only child. Jason has borne the brunt of what happened to Harvey and me. Alzheimer's has changed him too. How could it not? But this is not something either of us wants to discuss.

Lately, I have been trying to get my papers in order. Sorting through letters and mementos, I admonish myself not to be sentimental and toss them in the trash. Why leave curious and unanswered questions behind for Jason as Harvey did for me?

On my night shift, I take comfort in sitting alone in a living room surrounded by sentimental souvenirs we collected on our travels. There is no room on the coffee or side tables for even a drink. This is my memory shrine. It is the only place where my mind can go still. Many of the objects have small slips of paper underneath. My grandchildren are picking out—at my invitation—things they would love to have from Nana's collection. I am curious about what they treasure most and prefer to know now.

Hope sits in our kitchen taking endless photos of GG on her iPhone and recording their awkward attempts at conversation. Now fourteen years old, she is sensitive that just sitting with GG is the best way to connect. Her brother Eli, who just turned twelve, entertains us with a trumpet serenade while Benjamin, age nine, wheels himself past me in Grandpa Harvey's transport chair. This is how we make it through the holidays from one year to the next.

Dana and Jason have carefully coached them past their early fears. Over years we have built the lore of grandpa Harvey—athletic, full of fun, a special doctor and most of all, how much he would have loved and been proud of them. Researchers say our earliest memories fade by ages six to eight. It's not that we forget, but our brains aren't developed enough to retain them. But what happens to children who have to live face to face with Alzheimer's all their lives?

Alzheimer's creates a vacancy that cannot be filled. I want to enjoy being with those I love while I can still make memories with them.

A celebrated columnist asks me over dinner a question that has been troubling her: "Can you have true intimacy with another human being without shared memories?" She has started to write a column, but it remains unfinished, tucked away in a drawer. There is no easy answer to her question when you have lived the disease.

Everything I have done for my husband has been intimate, more than any adult would ever consider desirable. A caregiver must cross personal boundaries. The intimacy of total dependence and loss of control is one we all fear.

Over the years with Harvey, the care became clinical. I always took care of him with respect and love, but my attentions came without a hint of sexuality because Harvey cannot communicate either pleasure or gratitude. Shared memories must be built on both. Memories warm us. Separated from our memories, good or bad, who are we? In this sense, we have both lost out on an intimate life. But unlike Harvey, I still have memories that intensify my sense of loneliness. Long after the dinner with the columnist is over, I want to go back and offer her my answer. No. The answer is no. You cannot have intimacy with another human being without shared memories.

*Why are the walls in testing rooms always a dreary white, de*void of visual distractions? Why does the time between tests seem interminable? I am already starting to fret that I won't be able to remember the preceding battery of word associations when asked to recite the words back. Why can't I relax? Though tempted, I don't dare pick up my iPhone to check messages. I worry that I will lose focus and not perform well when the psychologist calls me back in. I do not want there to be a problem. Even more, I do not want the psychologist to notice I have a problem.

When Harvey became mute, so did I in many ways. When Tom Hutton, Trustee of the Geoffrey Beene Foundation, reached out, I found my voice again. It was a lifeline for which I will always honor him.

Every day I ask myself if I am doing anything that makes a difference. It surprises me a little that I am back taking the same kinds of tests Harvey once took. Doctors were the ones who kept telling me privately that Harvey couldn't last long. Their words strengthened my resolve to see him through to the end. But closure still seems far away.

The last of the husbands and wives with early-onset Alzhei- mer's in our small circle of care and support have all passed away. Their spouses—my friends—have moved on to recapture what's left of their lives; some more successfully than others. One man cannot erase the haunting image of his petite wife being carted off on a stretcher in a straightjacket from their upstairs bedroom in the middle of the night by police and medics. In their need to escape the past, they have stopped calling me. I understand and wish them well.

Strangers still reach out to commiserate and question me. For many, their journey with Alzheimer's has just begun. I make no pretense about having answers. Nonetheless, I am unable to brush aside their pain. I am a listener and sounding board more often than I am prescriptive.

• • •

After all that has happened, and given the unknown that lies ahead, I am still not sure that I could or even would have done things any differently.

I am a person who does not quit once she embarks on something important. There is a price to pay for that type of determination and I'm living it. I apply the same passion to my advocacy. I suppose that Alzheimer's is the final test of whether I can keep up such high standards for myself.

I make no assumptions about what I am doing. I replay constantly whether what I say or do will resonate in any way. I question whether telling my story will make any difference to anyone. Sometimes I think that greater public awareness about Alzheimer's, instead of reducing the ignorance and stigma, has actually increased it. Even those unlike Harvey, who announce defiantly to the world that they have early-onset Alzheimer's, are often marginalized professionally and later socially. A dementia-friendly society is not yet in reach.

There are academic scholars who argue that our fear of forgetting is irrational, a scare tactic of advocacy groups or businesses that want to sell anti-aging products. But I disagree. There is nothing irrational about our fear. Our fear matches the facts.

I worry that people will be offended by my honesty about this disease. I don't think I have done anything that other caregivers haven't done for family and friends they love—though perhaps I have done it longer. But I claim no special expertise, and I refuse to pretend that my way is the right way. My advocacy is all about making sure no one ends up like me.

Today has been emotionally exhausting and a bit unfulfilling. It is hard in this kind of study—stretching over years and years, the data not available to the participants—to truly feel that one is making a contribution. I long for a way to make research projects and trials more accessible to hundreds of thousands of us doing the same things over the years, all of us working together, a community of citizen scientists. I know that in time there will be an infusion of technology platforms that will make participation less cumbersome and the data more widely available to all who want to study it. Only then will we be able to reach the numbers of people needed to sustain prevention trials and long-term research.

The young researcher reenters the room and interrupts my conversation with myself. She politely asks if I am interested in giving a blood sample for a companion study. I defer apologetically. For now, I have tested my own limits. It is time to get back home.

It has been almost eight hours since I have checked in at home. The nurses knew that I would be offline, but they had the number to the testing lab in case of emergency. No urgent e-mails or text messages pop up on my screen. I check in anyway. After so many years, I can't imagine the feeling when I won't need to constantly check in—when I won't be needed in such a personal and intimate way. Is that what freedom from Alzheimer's will look like?

A few years ago, I read a study reporting that the public's second biggest fear, after getting Alzheimer's, is being a caregiver. I understand this feeling, and yet it is demoralizing. I became an advocate because I can't handle the pain any other way.

I've timed it right and arrive home just in time for the night shift. Grateful that Harvey and my mother have been put to bed a bit early, I listen to the nurse's report of the day. Harvey's vital signs are stable. He seems to be resisting nourishment, but it may just be getting more difficult for him to swallow without choking. We can only observe and guess. The nurses administer liquids through an eye dropper to hydrate him. My preference when on duty at night is to sip the liquid first, then softly kiss him, letting its wetness and warmth pass between us. When he opens his mouth for more, I like to imagine that it gives him pleasure but given the reality of the disease, I have no way to know. I do it anyway just in case.

Tonight I will shut out the light in the room for the first time in years. I used to leave it on to comfort him, but the doctors recently told me that his brain is shutting down. There is no fear left.

I undress, taking my place beside him, and whisper out loud. Would he be amused that I now share his passion for science, where before we lived in such separate worlds? Would he be proud that I have become such a strong supporter of researchers just like him, who never give up on their patients?

I thank him for being my teacher for all things that matter in life: love, loyalty, and family.

Harvey and I have been slow dancing with a stranger for years. Alzheimer's captured us both. It destroyed a wonderful mind and our life together. I have learned not to fight its strangle hold, but that has not stopped me from trying to escape it in other ways. Is it just a matter of time before I am next on its dance card?

When I stare in the mirror, I see only exhaustion and twenty years lost. I am still looking for the same thing I wanted when I first learned that Harvey had Alzheimer's disease: a way out for us all.

Am I repeating myself?

These days I rarely leave the house. I work by his bedside and keep up through conference calls. When I left in the morning for Boston, I kissed him, as I always do, as if it were the last time. I like to think we communicate through touch and that, even at this late stage in the disease, he can decode my messages of unconditional love. What I cannot hide in my touch is the enveloping and unspoken melancholy between us. I cannot save him.

. . .

I have no regrets that I insisted we do hospice at home or that I chose not to have strangers touch him in his waning days. If touch is the first sense we acquire, then I want the last touch he feels to be mine. I've earned it.

Acknowledgments

My story would never have made it to the printed page without the perseverance, patience, prodding and support of a number of individuals, who believed in its value to the national Alzheimer's dialogue and had confidence in my ability to tell it.

MY SINCERE APPRECIATION AND GRATITUDE

To my literary agent Will Lippincott, who called me the day after our story aired on PBS in August 2006 to encourage me to write a book. I resisted his thoughtful, yet persistent calls for five years. I am not sure either of us remembers exactly how or when he won me over.

To Gideon Weil, an inspiring Executive Editor at Harper One, who took a chance on a first time author; then nurtured and coached me through the entire editing and publishing process, even though I think that I am old enough to be his mother.

To Amy Dockser Marcus, a Pulitzer Prize–winning *Wall Street Journal* science and health reporter and personal friend, who offered caring, but critical feedback, and talked me through writer's block while challenging me to stay true to my narrative and lose the writing crutch of metaphors.

To Alun Davies, a revered figure in the publishing industry, who offered me insights into how his world works and honored me with a generous offer and masterful eye to read and critique my unfinished manuscript.

To Dr. Joseph G. Perpich, M.D., JD, psychiatrist and creator of the Virtual Collaboratory, whose eloquent notes on my manuscript will forever be cherished by this first time author.

To Harry Wade, a professional colleague and early collaborator, without whose assistance my original book proposal would still be languishing in a drawer somewhere.

To the entire team at HarperOne for their seamless support—Suzanne Wickham, Claudia Boutote, Mark Tauber, Hilary Lawson, Alison Petersen, and Jennifer Jensen.

HONORING OUR DONOR AND
CELEBRATING THE MISSION

To Tom Hutton, Trustee of the Geoffrey Beene Foundation and sole donor for the Geoffrey Beene Foundation Alzheimer's Initiative, for a generous opportunity of a lifetime to help make a difference in Alzheimer's awareness and early diagnosis.

To my dream team GBFAI Board, chaired by George Vradenburg and Dr. William Haseltine, who have advised and challenged me to seek out the most innovative and catalytic projects to advance our mission.

A special shout out to my colleagues at Geoffrey Beene, LLC who keep the vision and spirit of the legendary designer on the cutting edge of fashion and philanthropy.

TO THOSE ABOUT WHOM I CAN'T AND DIDN'T SAY ENOUGH

I could have written volumes about my family, friends, and colleagues who each deserved a chapter all their own.

To my family—Jason, Dana, Hope, Eli, and Ben, who are the sun, moon, and stars of my life. Thank you for your unwavering love and support and not giving Mom a hard time about sharing our very private journey with Alzheimer's on the chance it might be able to help others. For the record, the real author in our family is my daughter-in-law Dana, with five children's books and a novel, *A Year to Last a Lifetime*.

To Trish and George Vradenburg, who embrace me in their lives as an intimate friend, shore up my courage in tough times, and lead with unrelenting passion our fight to stop Alzheimer's by 2020.

To my glorious and talented women friends—Lisa Colburn, Michette Kapnist, Lin Arison, Judy Weiser, Ginny

Mancini, Jeanette Longoria, Rita Salzman, Rita Hortenstein, Bonnie Osher, Diane Perella, Arlene Herson, Florine Mark, Anastasia Beauscher, and Joan Challinor. Thank you for your loyalty, laughter, advice whether I ask or not, and open invitations to share your lives to underscore that I am not alone.

To the next generation philanthropists and spirited Alzheimer's advocates who will make their mark getting us to a cure: Leeza Gibbons, Karen Segal, Simone Friedman Rones, Lisa Spikell, and all the founding members of WomenAgainstAlzheimers.org.

And my personal gratitude and appreciation to all of you who cared enough personally or from a policy perspective to read this book and connect it with your own story or mission.

THE POWER OF US

USAgainstAlzheimers and its family of Networks:Women AgainstAlzheimer's, ResearchersAgainstAlzheimer's, African-AmericansAgainstAlzheimer's, HispanicsAgainstAlzheimer's, ClergyAgainstAlzheimer's, and ActivistsAgainstAlzheimer's.

About the Author

MERYL COMER, *an award-winning thirty-year veteran reporter*, producer, and talk show host, is President and CEO of the Geoffrey Beene Foundation Alzheimer's Initiative.

Comer was among the first TV newswomen in the 1980s to specialize in business news as it relates to public policy with a nationally syndicated debate show, *It's Your Business.* She also co-anchored *Nation's Business Today* for six years on ESPN and the ten o'clock news for Metromedia.

Winner of the 2005 Shriver Profiles in Dignity Award and the 2007 Proxmire Award, Ms. Comer has provided testimony before Congress, served on the 2008 Alzheimer's Study Group, and served two terms on the National Board of the Alzheimer's Association. She is a founding member of USAgainstAlzheimer's and cofounder of Women Against Alzheimer's Network.

In 2012, Comer led the formation of "The 21st Century BrainTrust™," a nonprofit alliance focused on wireless cognitive tracking and optimal brain health.

Comer has been the at-home caregiver for the past nineteen years for her husband with early-onset Alzheimer's disease and her mother with late-stage dementia. Her story has been profiled in the *The Washingtonian* and in *More* magazine and has been featured on *PBS NewsHour* and ABC *Nightline* with Terry Moran.

One hundred percent of proceeds from her book *Slow Dancing with a Stranger* will support Alzheimer's research.